D0017408

Live a Little Laugh a Lot

Barb Bancroft

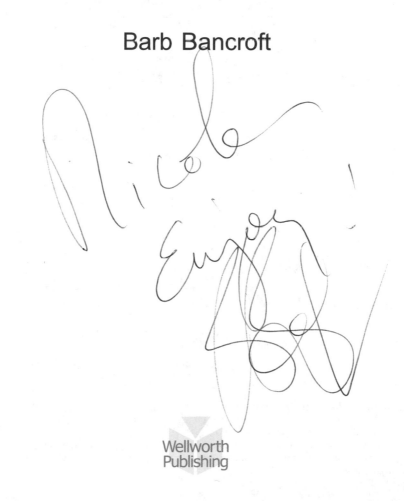

Wellworth
Publishing

Published by
WellWorth Publishing

Design and layout
Jean Sheldon

Illustrations
Ashley Long
Frank Salcido

Editor
Mary E. Harding

Library of Congress Control Number: 2003101948
ISBN 0-9723541-1-5

Printed in the United States of America

Copyright © 2003 Barb Bancroft
All rights reserved. Except for use in schools, educational institutions and non-profit agencies, the reproduction or use of this work in any form is forbidden without the written permission of the publisher.

> *The arrival of a good clown exercises a more beneficial influence on the health of a town than twenty asses laden with drugs.*
> —Dr. Thomas Sydenham (1624-1689)

Other Books by Barb Bancroft

Medical Minutiae

An Apple a Day–The ABCs of Diet & Disease

Bite Me
(Spring 2004)

Dedication

As always, to my Mom and Dad—parents extraordinaire. Without you, where would I be?

And, a special thank you to Dr. Barbara Brodie for providing me with the opportunity of a lifetime—to learn under your tutelage at the University of Virginia.

Acknowledgments

Four very special acknowledgments are in order here.

Jean Sheldon, computer whiz, graphic designer, humorist, critic, and friend…all rolled into one oingy-boingy package. We have collaborated on many things over the past 20 years, and with each experience you continue to amaze me with your broad knowledge base and expertise in all things dealing with the world of books, design and *computer-ease*. Thank you, Jean.

Rae Stith, for your ever-so-helpful critique of the cover design, tag lines, and complex layout of the book. Your way with words continues to astonish and amuse, and is most appreciated when I have reached an impasse on finding a word with more than one syllable. Many thanks, Raemond.

Mary Harding, my long-distance editor from Bemidji, Minnesota, also deserves a special acknowledgment. I am forever indebted to you for your continued willingness to edit not only my longer than long run-on sentences but also my lack of punctuation, too many em-dashes, not enough semi-colons, and an overabundance of elipses'. Thank you again, Mary.

Ashley Long, the fastest draw this side of the Mississippi. The rapidity with which you fire out those drawings is only eclipsed by your extraordinary talent as a cartoonist. I'm eagerly anticipating our next collaboration.

Table of Contents

Three to five minutes of belly laughing equals three minutes of strenuous exercise on a rowing machine.

(Toss the machine, and enjoy this book.)

Chapter 1

Live a Little, Laugh a Lot

> Doctors are whippersnappers in
>   ironed white coats
> Who spy up your rectums and look
>   down your throats.
> And press you and poke you with
>   sterilized tools,
> And stab at solutions that pacify
>   fools.
> I used to revere them and do what
>   they said
> Till I learned what they learned on
>   was already dead.
>
> —Gilda Radnor, 1988

Future health care professional "wanna-be's" have given the following answers to medical questions on high school biology tests. One can only hope that this particular group of students will succumb to the rigors of biochemistry and differential equations and be forced to choose another profession.

Q: "What is the best way to treat a nosebleed?"
A: "Put the nose much lower than the body until the heart stops."

Q: "What would you do for someone who has fainted?"
A: "Rub the person's chest, or, if a lady, rub her arm above the hand instead. Or put the head between the knees of the nearest medical doctor."

Q: "What is the definition of artificial insemination?"
A: "Artificial insemination is when the farmer does it to the cow instead of the bull."

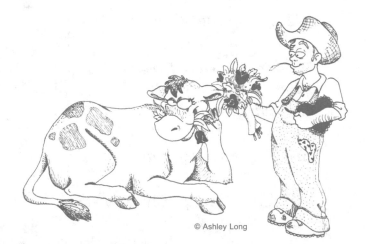

© Ashley Long

The search for intelligent life continues. During one of my too-numerous-to-count flights, an article in the TWA *Ambassador* magazine caught my eye and made me laugh right out loud. The article disclosed a list of questions posed to various visitor information bureaus throughout the U.S. Here are some of my favorites culled from the many included in the article.

Visitor's Bureau, Wine Country, Sonoma, California
"What are all of those dwarf trees all over those hills?"

Visitor's Bureau, Boise, Idaho
"If you go to a restaurant in Idaho and you don't want any kind of potato with your meal, will they ask you to leave?"

Visitor's Bureau, Salt Lake City, Utah
"What's the white stuff on top of the mountains? Is it salt?"

Visitor's Bureau, Anchorage, Alaska
"Do you have a map of the Iditarod trail? We would like to go for a walk now."

Visitor's Bureau, Philadelphia, Pennsylvania
"Where can I buy a picture of the Liberty Bell? In the one I have the bell has a crack in it."

Visitor's Bureau, Louisville, Kentucky
"If it rains, will the hot-air balloon race be held inside Freedom Hall?"

Visitor's Bureau, New Orleans, Louisiana
"How naked can you get at Mardi Gras? When is your next Jazz funeral?"

Visitor's Bureau, Pennsylvania Dutch Country
"Where can we find Amish hookers? We want to buy a quilt."

Visitor's Bureau, Florida Space Coast
"Which beach is the closest to the water?"

The search for intelligent life continues….

Would you want this geriatric physician for *your* surgeon? As reported in *USA Today* verbatim (September 21, 1996): A physician is being held without bail in San Diego, accused of killing a patient who died after his healthy leg was amputated. John Brown, 75, is accused of killing Philip Bondy, 80, who died in May of gangrene from an amputation performed in Tijuana. Bondy suffered from apotemnophilia, an overwhelming sexual desire to have a limb removed, the prosecutors said. Brown is also charged with practicing without a license. His California license was revoked in 1977 after three patients nearly died from sex-change operations he performed in a garage and a hotel.

Whoa. Still searching….

A smiley faced surgeon. Glenn Warden, chief surgeon at Cincinnati's Shriners' Burns Institute, was cleared in an ethics panel probe after he drew smiley faces on the genital areas of two patients. The hospital wouldn't comment on the probe, however, Warden stated that he drew "happy faces" on a 22-year-old man's genitals and on a woman's lower abdomen with their consent in order to relieve their tension about the surgical procedures.

Direct quotes from patient charts describing various clinical conditions:

• Healthy appearing, decrepit 90-year-old female, mentally alert, but forgetful.

• When she fainted, her eyes rolled around the room.

• Rectal exam revealed a normal-sized thyroid.

Live a Little, Laugh a Lot

- Examination of the genitalia was completely negative except for the right foot.

- Indwelling urinary catheter draining large amount of urine the color of American beer.

- History: Patient was shot in the head with a .32 caliber rifle. Chief complaint: Headache.

- Examination of the external genitalia reveals that he is circus-sized.

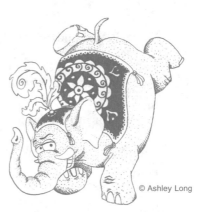
© Ashley Long

And what LIVE A LITTLE, LAUGH A LOT chapter would be complete without a list of attorney bloopers? The following questions were ripped from the pages of court reports and published in the *Massachusetts Bar Association Lawyers Journal*. These will answer any questions you might have about the stringent entrance requirements used by law schools to admit only the best and the brightest.

Q: "Now doctor, isn't it true that when a person dies in their sleep, they don't know about it until the next morning?"

Q: "Was it you or your younger brother who was killed in the war?"

Q: "How many times have you committed suicide?"

Q: "So, the date of conception (of the baby) was August 8th?"
A: "Yes."
Q. "And, what were you doing at the time?"

Q: "Doctor, how many autopsies have you performed on dead people?"
A: "All of my autopsies are performed on dead people."

Q: "Do you recall the time you examined the body?"

A: "The autopsy started around 8:30 p.m."

Q: "And Mr. Dennington was dead at the time?"

A: "No, he was sitting on the table wondering why I was doing an autopsy."

> *Lawyers are 3.6 times more likely to suffer depression than other professionals.*

Q: "All of your responses must be oral, OK?"

A: "Oral."

Q: "She had three children, right?"

A: "Yes."

Q: "How many were boys?"

A: "None."

Q: "Were there any girls?"

Q: "You were shot in the fracas?"

A: "No, I was shot midway between the fracas and the navel."

Q: "How far apart were the vehicles at the time of the collision?"

Written excuses from home. The following is a list of written excuses given to teachers in the Albuquerque Public School System by parents of students (May 1995). (Please note that the excuses are written exactly as they appeared.)

- Dear School: Please excuse John from being absent on January 28, 29, 30, 31, 32, and also 33.

- Please excuse Dianne from being absent yesterday. She was in bed with gramps.

- Please excuse Johnnie for being. It was his father's fault.

- Chris will not be in school because he has an acre in his side.

- John has been absent because he had two teeth taken off his face.

- Excuse Gloria. She has been under the doctor.

- Lillie was absent from school yesterday because she had a going over.

- My son is under the doctor's care and should not take fizical ed. Please execute him.

- Carlos was absent yesterday because he was playing football. He was hit in the growing part.

- My daughter was absent yesterday because she was tired. She spent the weekend with the Marines.

- Please excuse Joyce from PE for a few days. Yesterday she fell off a tree and misplaced her hip.

- Please excuse Ray Friday from school. He has very loose vowels.

- Maryann was absent December 11-16, because she had a fever, sore throat, headache, and upset stomach. Her sister was also sick, fever and sore throat, her brother had a low-grade fever. There must be the flu going around, her father even got hot last night.

- Please excuse Blanche from jim today. She is administrating.

- George was absent yesterday because he had a stomach.

- Ralph was absent yesterday because he had a sore trout.

- Please excuse Sara for being absent. She was sick and I had her shot.

- Please excuse Lupe. She is having problems with her ovals.

- Please excuse Pedro from being absent yesterday. He had diah (crossed out), diahoah (crossed out), dyah (crossed out) the shits.

The search continues....

Comments from patients during rectal exams (James Ralph, MD):

"Take it easy, Doc—you're boldly going where no man has gone before."

"Find Amelia Earhart yet?"

"Can you hear me NOW?"

"Oh boy, that was sphincteriffic!"

"Could you write me a note for my wife, saying that my head is not, in fact, up there?"

"You know, in some states, we're now legally married."

"Any sign of the trapped miners, Chief?"

"You put your left hand in, you take your left hand out, you do the hokey pokey."

"Hey! Now I know how a muppet feels."

"If your hand doesn't fit, you must acquit!"

"Hey Doc, let me know if you find my dignity."

"Remind me never to become an altar boy."

"You used to be an executive at Enron, didn't you?"

"Are we there yet? Are we there yet? Are we there yet?"

"How long have you been in politics?"

"Been there, done that!!!"

Golf balls and pesticides. In the British gastroenterology journal, cleverly named *Gut,* a golfer was referred to a GI specialist for unexplained abdominal pains and lethargy. Upon taking a thorough history, it was revealed that the golfer would lick his golf ball in order to clean it and give it a quick spit shine. This procedure over time resulted in the accumulation of toxic amounts of pesticide residue, resulting in the aforementioned symptoms. His symptoms miraculously disappeared when he switched from using his tongue to using a damp rag to clean his balls, so to speak.

Golf courses, toxic chemicals, cigars. Well, apparently golf balls aren't the only carriers of pesticide residue. If a golfer lays his cigar on the putting green or any other part of the golf course prior to hitting the ball, it may become contaminated with the pesticides and herbicides sprayed on the golf course to kill the unwanted weeds and irritating insects. Reports of flocks of geese that died shortly after landing and walking on recently sprayed golf courses revealed that their bodies were toxic with lawn chemicals.

So, for those of you who are cigar-chompin' golfers, heed this warning and take this advice. Purchase a cigar holder, made expressly for the purpose of reducing golf course toxicity, and use it every time you need to use both hands to swing the club. And, since most golf course chemicals tend to be so toxic, it may be wise to avoid playing on the days that the course has been freshly sprayed. You can also minimize contact with these chemicals by washing your hands and arms immediately after playing, wearing long pants instead of shorts, not walking barefoot on the course, and by never holding tees in your mouth, or as cited above, using your tongue to clean your golf balls. (*The Physician and Sportsmedicine*, 1998; 26(2):18)

Kissin' and itchin'. A group of physicians in Naples, Italy reported on an unusual case of oral transmission of allergies. A woman's husband was taking ampicillin for a mouth infection and she proceeded to kiss her husband in a passionate way. Shortly afterwards she suffered from itching and swelling of the lips and throat. She reported that she had suffered similar symptoms after taking the same antibiotic for an infection four years earlier. The physicians, trained to be skeptics, worked her up for every allergy known to man and concluded after seven months that it must have been the kiss. But, to prove their point, they gave the husband antibiotic pills or placebo pills on different days and "ordered" him to kiss his wife. Well, the conclusion to the story is obvious. On the days that he took the antibiotics she developed swelling and itching and on the days that she received placebo-only kisses she had no allergic reaction. Needless to say, oral transmission of a drug allergy is quite rare, but it happens. (*Lancet*, 2002)

Kissin' relatives. Every once in awhile a newspaper story catches my eye. Since many of my readers have more important things to do besides read *USA Today* (where I get all of my clinical information), I will often share the stories with my students, seminar participants, and faithful newsletter subscribers. Here's one that caught my eye and in turn, elicited a huge guffaw.

Police in central Florida discovered that farmhand Samuel Patrick 52, and his sister Debra, 44, had nine children together while cohabiting as husband and wife. Samuel Patrick was arrested for incest. A police spokeswoman won the prize for the best quote after this story surfaced in the news. She said "Not *all* the kids look funny."

Kissin' cousins. Well, if marrying your sister is out of the question, can you marry your cousin and have a perfectly healthy, normal child? Yes and no, with a heavy emphasis toward the *no*. Even though the risk of having a child with birth defects is *lower* than previously believed, first and second cousins who decide to tie the knot are still more likely to have children with mental retardation, birth defects, or a recessive genetic disease. An unrelated couple has a 3 to 4 percent chance of having a child with such problems whereas a related couple has a 5 to 8 percent chance depending on the disease. Recessive diseases such as cystic fibrosis and Tay-Sachs disease have a much greater chance of being passed on in first cousin marriages. Five to eight percent doesn't sound like a lot, but let's put it this way—a 7 to 8 percent chance of a genetic disorder is 50 percent greater than a 5 percent chance, so why take the chance? Expand your horizons! Move out of Possum Holler and meet someone that doesn't have your same last name! In fact, in 30 states in the U.S. it's *illegal* to marry your cousin Betty Sue Hatfield or Jimmy Joe McCoy. But if you insist, California, Wyoming, Colorado, New Mexico, Texas, Louisiana, Wisconsin, Tennessee, Alabama, Florida, South Carolina, Virginia, West Virginia, Michigan, New York, New Jersey, Connecticut, and Vermont still allow first cousin marriages. Geneticists estimate that one in every 1,000 marriages in the U.S. is between first cousins. Anyone want to take a wild stab as to which state has the most?

Most Western cultures find this practice to be undesirable; however, this practice is still acceptable some cultures in Africa, Asia, and the Middle East including Saudi Arabia and Pakistan. Jewish and Christian religions discourage the practice and the Roman Catholic Church requires cousins to get permission before they marry. (*Journal of Genetic Counseling,* April 2002)

Hospital admissions on weekends—stay home if at all possible. It appears as if hospital admissions on weekends are much more hazardous to your health than if admission occurs during the week. Researchers in Ontario looked at 100 of the most common causes of death and found that for 23 of them, the risk of death was significantly greater if patients went to the hospital on a weekend. All 100 conditions were more likely to be fatal on weekends. Among the conditions more likely to be fatal on the weekend: ruptured aorta in the abdomen, 41 percent vs. 36 percent on weekdays; pulmonary embolism, 13 percent vs. 11 percent; and kidney failure, 36 percent vs. 30 percent. Why are weekend admissions more dangerous? Ever worked a weekend? Doesn't take a rocket scientist to figure out why…one RN for 3,398 patients…in other words, low staffing is most likely the "pathogen." (*N Engl J of Med* 30 August 2001;345(9):663-8)

Leaving "things" behind in the operating room. Well, I guess it wouldn't be that funny if it happened to you, but it appears as if your surgery is an emergency, surgeons are more likely to leave a memento

> *Half of the surgical sponges left in patients remain undiscovered for a period of five or more years after surgery.*

behind—clamps, forceps, sponges, electrodes, and the like. In fact, if your surgery is an emergency surgery, the likelihood is *nine* times more likely. (Harvard School of Public Health, January 2003)

Murphy's Law has its origins from U.S. Air Force studies performed in 1949. Captain Edward A. Murphy designed a harness to monitor the effects of rapid deceleration on pilots. Volunteers were strapped on a rocket-propelled sled, and their condition was monitored as the sled was brought to an abrupt halt. The harness designed by Murphy worked flawlessly on the first day; however, in a subsequent test to validate the initial findings the harness failed to record any data whatsoever. Murphy discovered that every single electrode had been wired incorrectly. Frustrated by the error, Captain Murphy declared, "If there were two or more ways of doing something, and one of them can lead to catastrophe, then someone will do it." Before long—and much to Murphy's chagrin—his principle was soon transformed into an apparently flippant statement about day-to-day misfortunes. In other words, "Why do I always pick the longest check-out line at Target?" or "Why do I always get the behind the guy with the Pitney-Bowes machine at the post office?" Murphy's Law, that's why.

SHIT (Ship High in Transport). In the sixteenth and seventeenth centuries, everything had to be transported by ship. It was also before commercial fertilizer's invention, so large shipments of manure were common. It was shipped dry, because in dry form it weighed quite a bit less than in wet form. However, once the seawater hit the dry manure, it not only became heavier, but the process of fermentation began again, the by-product of which is methane gas.

As the stuff was stored below the decks in bundles the methane built up in the enclosed space. The first time someone moseyed on down into the lower decks with a lantern, KABOOM! Several ships were destroyed in this manner. After that, the bundles were always stamped with the term Ship High in Transit, which meant for the sailors to stow it high enough off the lower decks so that any water that came into contact with it would not start the production of methane.

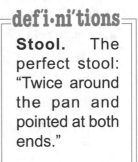

def'i·ni'tions

Stool. The perfect stool: "Twice around the pan and pointed at both ends."

The toilet bowl as a diagnostic tool. Four hundred years ago Dr. Thomas Willis suggested that urine could be used to diagnose illnesses in patients. In fact, he believed that tasting the urine would be the most accurate way to determine the cause of various signs and symptoms in his patient population. He was the first physician to diagnose "the sweet taste of the urine" and to recognize the quick deterioration of the patient once the urine was sweet.

Now, most nurses and physicians weren't too keen on slugging down a cup of urine, however in the 1600s this was accepted practice. Actually just a taste would suffice. If the urine tasted like sugar it was diagnosed as diabetes mellitus. Diabetes means 'to siphon' and mellitus means 'sweet'. If the patient's urine had absolutely no taste, it was called diabetes insipidus. Insipid means tasteless, in other words it tasted just like water. Times changed, urine was no longer accepted as a beverage so if a patient came into the physician's office and said, "Doc, I'm peein' too much," the urine sample would be collected and placed on the back porch of the doctor's office. After ten minutes the nurse would stick her head out of the door and check the urine sample. If there were bees, ants or flies around it the urine contained sugar—hence, the name diabetes mellitus. If the urine had no bugs in the immediate vicinity the patient most likely had diabetes insipidus. Either way, whether it was a quick slug of the urine or whether it was placed on the back porch, the testing of urine was cost effective.

Crapper, Thomas. An English sanitary engineer, invented the first flush lavatory, known as Crapper's Valveless Water Waste Preventor in 1837. The word *crap* is derived from the crapper.

Clinical help for nondiseases. What are the top "problems" people seek help for that are really *not* considered to be diseases?

1) Getting old
2) Baldness
3) Jet lag
4) Road rage
5) Loneliness
6) Boredom (see below)
7) Anxiety about penis size (I realize that this deserves a comment, but I just can't do it. I want to, but just can't.) (*British Medical Journal*, April 2002)

Bored? Check out The Boring Institute, P.O. Box 40, Maplewood NJ 07040. Be sure to fork over $12.50 for the guide, *Ten Secrets to Avoid Boredom.*

Occupational hazard of monks. Monks from yesteryear must have spent an inordinate time on their knees—praying at midnight, praying at sunrise, praying twice during the day, at sunset, and again before bedtime. One monk, from a Byzantine monastery around 500 A.D. wrote about his nightly practice of descending 18 steps into the holy cave and making 100 genuflections with each step. Susan Sheridan, an anthropologist from Notre Dame, studied 6,000 skeletal remains from the aforementioned monastery and found that their general health was quite robust. However, their kneecaps were worn to a frazzle. She observed the characteristic roughening of arthritis at the points where the muscles used in kneeling attach to the bone and concluded that the major occupational hazard of monks was arthritis of the knees.

Occupational hazard of church bell ringers. Lightning is considered to be quite an occupational hazard of church bell ringers. In the Middle Ages it was common practice to ring church bells to dispense with thunder. This practice was not very successful for many reasons—the most obvious being that it didn't work. However, the success rate of a lightning bolt hitting a bell tower was quite high. When lightning struck the bell tower it most often took the ringer right along with it.

Occupational hazard of coroners. Chuck West, a coroner in Kane County, Illinois reports that his office has had to invest in hydraulic equipment and larger storage facilities to handle the number of obese "clients." In the last 18 months, West's office has had seven corpses that weighed more than 500 pounds each. On each of the occasions they have had to call the fire department to help them move the corpse.

Occupational hazard of morticians. The January 27, 2000 issue of the *New England Journal of Medicine* reported the first documented case of cadaver to mortician transmission of tuberculosis (TB). The researchers compared the DNA "fingerprints" of the TB in both patients and found the exact same type of TB. The only time the two individuals had been exposed to each other was during the embalming process, when the blood was removed from the deceased, and the embalming fluids were injected to preserve the body. The embalmer most likely inhaled the infectious particles, probably created from the frothing of fluids through the nose and mouth of the deceased. This discovery helps to explain why funeral home workers have had higher rates of TB infection and disease than the general population.

Occupational hazard of working in a crematorium. Pacemakers have a nasty propensity to explode during cremation. The pacemakers contain combustible materials that can suddenly explode, endangering the crematorium workers. Over half of the 241 British crematoriums have reported explosions, some of which were strong enough to blow the doors off the crematorium ovens. Yikes.

Occupational hazard of being a chimney sweep. Here's one that will knock your knickers right off. London has been long famous for its smog and soot. In the eighteenth century chimney sweeps were slight young men who spent their day covered in soot. Bathing wasn't a priority and the young chimney sweeps could go, and would go, for months without bathing. Well, as it turns out, one of the consequences of long-term soot covering the body from the tip of the nose to the tip of the toes was scrotal cancer. And so, chimney sweeps were the number one risk group for this rather unique malignancy.

Dr. Percival Pott, a physician in London, was well aware of the risks of scrotal cancer in chimney sweeps. He actually wrote a book in the mid-eighteenth century about the occupational hazards of many groups, one of course, being the chimney sweep. He also declared at the time that if the chimney sweeps would consider *washing* their bodies just once a week (that's all he asked, was just once a week), this particular malignancy could be prevented. And lo and behold, he was right. Chimney sweeps scrubbed that scrotal cancer right off with weekly baths. So Dr. Percival Pott was one of the first physicians to recommend the simple procedure known as *bathing* as a public health measure to prevent a disease—and a malignancy at that. If all malignancies were that simple to prevent and cure, the word cancer would be relegated to a historical highlight.

> ## Historical Highlights
> During the Middle Ages the Celts perfected a method for making soap for the masses. This method spread throughout much of Europe, but many people feared that bathing too frequently—more than once a month, or in some regions, more than once a year—could be dangerous to one's health, if not fatal.

Occupational hazard of working in a dentist's office. An occupation hazard for thousands of female dentists, dental hygienists, and dental assistants is the exposure to laughing gas, also known as nitrous oxide. A study from the National Institute of Environmental Health in Research Triangle Park, N.C. (1993), found that dental hygienists with five or more hours of exposure to high levels of nitrous oxide per week were only 41 percent as likely as their peers to conceive each month. Women who were exposed to lower levels of gas (for example, dental offices with excellent ventilation) had normal fertility rates. In other words, women who were not exposed to nitrous oxide because of adequate ventilation took an average of six months to conceive. Women who worked with high levels of nitrous oxide in nonvented environments took an average of 32 menstrual cycles to conceive. The researchers postulated that nitrous oxide blocks secretion of gonadotropin-releasing hormone from the hypothalamus. This, in turn, blocks FSH (follicle stimulating hormone) and LH (luteinizing hormone), and disrupts the development of the ovarian follicle and subsequent ovulation. One other possible mechanism is that nitrous oxide may interrupt the normal process of maturation of the fertilized egg and thus cause a very early miscarriage.

Hey guys, women may not be the only gender with fertility problems. Researchers from Vancouver, British Columbia, have demonstrated that nitrous oxide has been shown to produce abnormalities in sperm as well as reduced fertility—but only in laboratory rats thus far.

Occupational hazard of hairdressers. Frequent exposure to hair spray and perming chemicals slightly increases the likelihood of a woman giving birth to a child with a low birth weight, heart defect, cleft palate, cleft lip, spina bifida, or other birth defects. (University Hospital, Lund, Sweden 2000)

Occupational hazards of hospital hairdressers. It appears as if Hortense, the hospital hairdresser, just might be the Typhoid Mary of MRSA (methicillin-resistant staphylococcus aureus). In a study reported in the *Journal of Hospital Infections* (November 2001; 49: 225-7), researchers traced an outbreak of MRSA to the hospital hairdresser and her contaminated hairdressing tools. It appears as if infection control policies in most hospitals don't require adequate decontamination of these tools and cross-infection can occur readily between patients. And, most likely the hospital hairdresser acquired the infection from one of her patients.

Occupational hazard of the long-distance runner. The die-hard long-distance runner is at high risk for the development of gallstones. This is presumably a consequence of chronic intravascular hemolysis from red blood cell damage from running. Also these individuals are at risk for iron deficiency anemia, basically for the same reason. The constant pounding on the pavement results in microscopic bleeding into the tissues. This in turn causes a loss of iron and a resultant iron deficiency anemia.

Scientists recently tested strands of hair reputed to be snipped from Napoleon's locks. They found arsenic levels that were about 35 times higher than normal and they concluded that Napoleon must have died from arsenic poisoning.

Occupational hazard of Bronze Age metal workers. Arsenic was probably the first substance banned as an occupational hazard. As long as 5,000 years ago, Bronze Age metal workers stopped smelting arsenic because of its adverse side effects which included pain, numbness, and weakness in the legs. This explains why the Greek, Roman, and Germanic gods of metalworking were all portrayed as lame.

Occupational hazards of felt hat workers. Mercury was once used in the silvering of mirrors and in the production of felt hats. The felt hat workers often developed toxic central nervous system changes, called madness, hence the phrase, "mad as a hatter," described by Lewis Carroll in *Alice in Wonderland*.

Recreational hazards of sitting in saunas. It doesn't matter what time of the year it is—if you have coronary artery disease (angina or a history of a myocardial infarction), stay out of saunas. Researchers at the Montreal Heart Institute in Quebec have found that individuals with angina have a high risk for a myocardial infarction when soaking in a sauna. The heat of the sauna increases the heart rate, and diminishes blood flow to the arteries that supply the heart, thus increasing the possibility of a myocardial infarction. (*Am J of Medicine*, September 1999)

Recreational hazard of deer hunting. Of course you can't shovel snow because of the risk of a heart attack (see next page), but don't think you can talk your wife into letting you go deer hunting because it's safer.

Frequent reports correlating deer hunting with myocardial infarctions and sudden cardiac death triggered a group of cardiologists at

William Beaumont Hospital in Royal Oak, Michigan to study the cardiac effects of deer hunting. They put cardiac monitors on ten deer hunters with established cardiovascular disease just to get a picture of heart health during the hunting season.

Measured against maximum heart rates on treadmill tests, just traipsing through the woods resulted in heart rates that were significantly higher than the normal heart rate. Other activities that contributed to higher heart rates included just seeing a deer, shooting and missing the deer, and the highest heart rates of all were when the hunter shot and hit the deer. The higher the heart rate, the higher the risk of heart attacks, hence, deer hunting can be hazardous to one's cardiovascular health, especially if heart disease is already established.

> *The trouble with heart disease is that the first symptom is often hard to deal with: sudden death.*
> Michael Phelps, M.D.

Seasonal hazards of shoveling snow. I'll start with the bottom line: Don't do it if you have a history of heart disease or if you are at high risk for heart disease. Researchers from William Beaumont Hospital in Royal Oak, Michigan collected data on sudden cardiac deaths around the time of two winter storms in 1999 and 2000. Of the 43 who expired after physical exertion, 36 had been shoveling snow near the time of their death. Lifting heavy, wet snow raises heart rates and blood pressures to the maximum levels of cardiac treadmill tests. Cold temperatures increase cardiovascular danger by further raising blood pressure, and chilly air decreases the amount of blood that can get to the heart. (*J Am Col Cardiology* March 6, 2002)

Ok, ok, ok, so you *have* to shovel the driveway. You live in Buffalo, New York, there's 62 inches of snow in the driveway and there's absolutely no getting around it if you ever want to leave the house in the winter. Here are a few helpful hints to avoid a heart attack:

1) Wait at least one to two hours after waking up before you start shoveling. You have an increased risk of having a heart attack

in the early morning because of physiologic factors such as an increased ability to clot combined with the increased workload of the heart upon arising.

2) Walk or stretch for 5 to15 minutes before starting the chore.

3) Use a small, lightweight shovel blade so that you lift lighter loads and therefore put less stress on the heart.

Monday morning heart attacks. A study of 2,636 patients hospitalized for myocardial infarctions revealed that the risk of having a heart attack for a blue-collar worker is 41 percent higher on Monday mornings than any other day of the week. For white-collar workers the risk is 18 percent higher on Mondays. The study also confirmed previous research that myocardial infarctions occur three times more frequently in the morning than any other time of the day.

Risky business—holidays! It is a well-established fact that heart attacks occur more frequently in the early morning hours, Monday especially. This peak incidence is attributed to an increase in catecholamines (the hormones of stress known as epinephrine, norepinephrine and dopamine) with the resultant increased workload of the heart as well as the increase in clotting factors in the early morning.

A lesser-known fact is that heart attacks occur in a seasonal pattern as well. A research team from UCLA examined the month-by-month death rate from myocardial infarctions over a 12-year period. They found that it stayed relatively stable through November and then increased dramatically after Thanksgiving and peaked around New Year's Day. The incidence of heart attacks increased by 33 percent in December and January.

One would perhaps assume that the winter trigger for heart attacks would be the cold weather and subsequent coronary vasoconstriction resulting in an increased workload of the heart. However, upon closer scrutiny, one discovers that the study was done in Southern California where the temperatures rarely dip below 50 degrees Fahrenheit, even on the coldest day of the year. One theory circles the drain.

The second traditional theory blames the good old American way of overindulging during the holiday season—lots of booze, fatty foods, and salt to make the season bright. This makes perfectly good sense in that all of the above work as a unit to overwork the heart during the most stressful season of the year.

A third theory has recently been proposed. This theory is based on cardiovascular changes due to biorhythm disturbances. Researchers at the Krannert Institute of Cardiology in Indianapolis speculate that the brain's biological clock may respond to short daylight hours in winter by altering the production of catecholamines (stress hormones) and cortisol. These stress hormones not only increase the workload of the heart, making it pump harder and faster, but they also increase the ability of platelets to stick to fat plaques in the vessels and subsequently trigger the clotting cascade.

P.S. Were any of you wondering what the *lowest-risk* months for heart attacks are in the U.S.? The answer is June and September with July and August coming in a close third and fourth.

Wedding bands and arthritis. A study in the December 1998 *Annals of the Rheumatic Diseases* found an interesting relationship between wearing a wedding ring and the development of arthritis. Of 55 patients with rheumatoid arthritis for at least two years, the 30 who wore gold bands had significantly less erosion of the second joint of the left finger than of the same joint on the right hand. The ring wearers also had less erosion in the joints of the left little and middle fingers. In the remaining 25 patients who had not worn rings, there was no difference between the left and right ring-finger joints. Of course, this wedding band remedy doesn't do much for the big picture of rheumatoid arthritis when multiple joints have aches and pains. *Hardly* enough of a reason to get married would you say?

Attention Shoppers!! Anti-theft devices may be hazardous to your health—especially if you have implanted defibrillators. The anti-theft devices may trigger the defibrillator to kick in, believing that an arrhythmia has developed. Be aware of this possibility when shopping, especially if a fellow shopper suddenly drops to the floor near an anti-theft device. If this happens, gently pull the patient away from the doors and the devices and observe to make sure their heart kicks back in.

Stress tests and security systems. If you have recently had an exercise stress test using a substance known as thallium you may set off security systems from Wal-Mart to the White House. Take a letter from your cardiologist with you if you are going anywhere within a few hours of a stress test—the airport comes to mind.

How do you recognize an adult who has been breast-fed? March right up to the suspect and palpate the tip of his or her nose. The nose will feel as if there are two separate cartilages underlying your finger. In sucklings (the oh-so British term for children who breast feed), the physical effects of breast pressure result in the two nasal cartilages being kept separate. In bottle-fed children the nasal cartilages unite and present in the adult as a single sharp outline. (Gill D, O'Brien N. *Pediatric Clinical Examination.* 3rd Edition, 1998. Churchill-Livingstone, London, UK)

Philtrum. This is the anatomic name for that little indentation that runs down under the nose to the upper lip and catches "snot" on the way out of the nostrils. Almost every animal has a philtrum—even lizards. Actually the philtrum is made from two ridges that are "sewn" together *in utero* to close up the two sides of the face. The ridges are actually there for a reason. They protect a particularly sensitive spot in the skull where three bones meet— two from the sides and one from the top. (The one from the top is the one that keeps the nostrils separate.) If the ridges fail to develop in the human, the child is born with a cleft lip

The word *philtrum* is actually derived from the Greek word, *philtron,* meaning 'love charm'. The ancient Greeks thought that the lips resembled the shape of Cupid's bow. The philtrum then, metaphorically represented the grip, the center of Cupid's power.

Head shape and snoring. Well, it might not be too late. You might be able to pick out a snoreless partner 75 percent of the time if you scrutinize their head shape before you fall madly in love and can't live without them. Look for someone with an oval head, not a round head.

Individuals with round heads have shorter throats and are prone to sleep apnea and chronic snoring. Individuals with rounder heads have rounder faces versus those with oval heads and thinner, elongated faces. Hmmmm…take a look at your significant other and see if it's too late to make your decision. You probably don't even need to look—you have heard it all night, every night, for 25 years.

> *Giving birth is like trying to push a piano through a transom.*
> —Alice Roosevelt Longworth (1884-1980)

So the best you can do, at this point, is to pass this information along to friends who are currently looking for Mr. or Ms. Right. Researchers at Case Western Reserve University compared head shapes of 60 snorers to 60 non-snorers. Using radiographic techniques they created a "craniofacial risk index" by measuring the size of the neck, airways and shape of the head. As the head gets relatively wider, the airway becomes relatively narrower from front to back. An unbiased researcher was able to predict sleep apnea problems three out of four times by using the craniofacial index.

So, can you differentiate sleep apnea from just plain old snoring? The common sleep disorder known as sleep apnea can be diagnosed with a simple home tape recording. The person with sleep apnea has characteristic snorts and snores that can be distinguished easily from the routine snorers. As the patient with sleep apnea progresses through the various stages of sleep, they may stop breathing for up to 20 seconds. This "apnea" is followed by a partial reawakening with a gasping snort for oxygen. This cycle is repeated throughout the night with the final result being a lousy night of oxygen-deprived sleep. Research has shown that long-term problems with sleep apnea can result in high blood pressure and/or coronary heart disease.

Diagnosing sleep apnea in the past has been rather costly because it required a night or two in an expensive sleep disorder laboratory. However, a group of researchers from the Sleep Disorders Center at St. Louis University tested a cheaper alternative. Based on the knowledge that the cartoonish snorts, snores, clucks, and hrumpfs of sleep apnea are distinctive, the researchers asked the partners of 50 problem snorers to make a home recording of their dearly beloved snoring significant other. The researchers then listened to the tapes to make the diagnosis. The 50 snorers then spent the night in the sleep disorder lab to verify the findings on the homemade tape recordings. Sleep apnea was correctly identified by the home recordings more than 90 percent of the time.

Patients with obstructive sleep apnea tend to have short, stocky necks. Many of these patients wear unusually large-collared shirts (greater than size 17), and still leave them unbuttoned. (Shapira, JD. *The Art and Science of Bedside Diagnosis.* Williams and Wilkins, Baltimore, 1990)

Speaking of short stocky necks. A recent study determined that in addition to being pulverized every Sunday in the fall and early winter, a second major occupational hazard of linemen in the National Football League (NFL) is sleep apnea. Check out their head shape and their body size—it's a no brainer. As many as 34 percent of the massive offensive and defensive lineman have sleep apnea, according to a study in the *New England Journal of Medicine,* 23 January 2003; 348 (4): 367-8.

Snooze alarms. How often do you slap that snooze alarm button on the top of the clock radio by the bed in the morning? *USA Today* reports that over one-third of the adult population pounds unmercifully on that button for an extra few minutes of blissful sleep every morning. In fact, the average number of hits every morning is three. It also appears as if the reliance on the snooze alarm is age-specific. Fifty-seven percent of the 25- to 34-year-old age group depends on the snooze alarm whereas only 10 percent of those over 65 regularly hit the button.

The loudest recorded snore on record is 87.5 decibels. This is the average decibel level of an alarm clock.

Snorgasms—the malady of marriages. Dr. David Schnarch, the director of the Marriage and Family Health Center in Evergreen, Colorado, reports that boredom and low sexual desire easily top the list of gripes among married couples seeking counseling. One of the most common complaints involves husbands falling asleep immediately after orgasm. In fact, this condition is so common, therapists have coined the term *snorgasm* for this postcoital predisposition.

Snoring. An otolaryngologist at the University of Minnesota suspended a microphone 24 inches above the heads of 1,139 sleeping men and women. He found that snoring that exceeded 49 decibels indicated a high risk of sleep apnea. Overweight individuals and men snored the loudest with 12 percent of the subjects topping 55 decibels, roughly the loudness of rush-hour traffic. Patients who have sleep apnea have a high risk of developing hypertension, arrhythmias, stroke, coronary heart disease, depression, memory loss and erectile dysfunction.

Snoring and relationships. A study by Bruskin/Goldring for Mission Pharmacal found that one in three adults has a partner who snores and that snoring has the following effect on relationships: 52 percent of the partners just hear "white noise" because it's been so long; 15 percent are grouchy in the morning; 11 percent leave the room and sleep in another bedroom or on the couch; 6 percent decided that if you can't beat 'em, join 'em, and started snoring too; and 11 percent reported miscellaneous effects. (Quantum Sufficit, *American Fam Physician* 1998; 58(6):1277)

So you think you're sleeping alone? After collecting dust samples from beds in 800 homes, U.S. government researchers found dust mite droppings in excess of 2 mg per gram of dust, a level known to trigger allergies in 44 million homes. In half of these homes they were fivefold higher—enough to keep you wheezin' and sneezin' for the next century. So—what to do? Turn that humidifier on, wash those sheets in scalding water, and zip up those duvet covers and pillows in allergy-proof covers. Whew! You're safe again…oops…not so fast. The U.S. government researchers also found another friend in bed with you—cockroaches and their excrement are present in approximately 6 million. And, cockroaches with their dander and their excrement are also potent allergens. An allergist from Harvard Medical School has reported that up to 50 percent of the allergic individuals in the Boston area who are exposed to roaches will develop an allergic sensitivity to the pesky critters. Roach fact: For every one roach you find in your house, scurrying across the kitchen counter, there are 800 to 2,000 hiding. According to a team of cockroach counters from the Agricultural Research Center in Gainesville Florida, 97.5 percent of 1,000 low-income apartments are infested with a minimum of 160 roaches per dwelling (RPD), with an average of 33,600 roaches per dwelling and up to 250,000 roaches per dwelling in the worst case scenario. You'll never sleep alone, again. (American Lung Association/American Thoracic Society Meeting 2000)

Fish tanks, diseases and salvaging marriages. A survey by the American Pet Products Manufacturers Association concluded that fish owners are not only much healthier than non-fish owners but they have happier marriages as well. Fish owners have less heart disease, less high blood pressure, less depression, less stress, fewer headaches, and they are more likely to drink less (if at all) and eat less. In addition they have fewer fights with their spouses and are less likely to have fits of jealousy. Hmmmm…is there a fish in your future? (Quantum Sufficit. *American Family Physician* 1998; 59(7):1729)

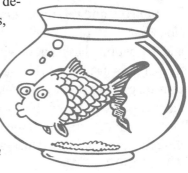

An unusual cause for a stuffy nose. Goeran Rudolfsson was plagued by nasal congestion after undergoing cranial surgery for a brain tumor. After blowing his nose one day he sensed a peculiar fullness in one nostril and gently reached into the nasal passage to determine the cause of the fullness. He was able to grasp a foreign object and he proceeded to pull out a 31-inch-long piece of gauze that had been placed in his head during the surgery to absorb fluids. A member of the operating team forgot to remove this piece of material when the procedure was completed. His chronic nasal congestion was miraculously cured.

Another possible cause of a stuffy nose. A small study in the Netherlands found that people suffering from chronic sinusitis have low amounts of glutathione, an antioxidant compound found in fruits and vegetables such as watermelon, grapefruit, oranges, asparagus, potatoes, and broccoli. The glutathione contained in these foods may assist in keeping free radicals in check in the linings of the upper respiratory tract. Keeping free radicals in check may reduce the chronic inflammation associated with sinusitis. Wouldn't hurt to give it a try if you're one of those plagued with the problem.

Swallowing pennies. If your kids are into swallowing pennies, make sure that they swallow the pennies minted prior to 1982. For almost 200 years our favorite coin was made of either pure or nearly pure copper. But in 1982, the U.S. Mint, ever mindful of the rising costs of copper, changed the composition of the coin to 97.5 percent zinc and 2.5 percent copper.

Unfortunately this combination can lead to a problem when swallowed by unsuspecting toddlers. The stomach acid (pH 2) can demolish the copper coating of the coins dated after 1982 within 24 hours. The zinc inside the coin reacts with the stomach acid to form hydrogen gas and zinc chloride. This chemical reaction is similar to the one that occurs in zinc-sulfuric acid batteries and can lead to gastric erosion, penetrating gastric ulcers and systemic reactions due to zinc toxicity.

An FYI concerning pennies. In 1943 pennies were made of steel and were zinc-covered. This was due to a shortage of copper during this critical war year. So, if you're a coin collector with kids, hide these zinc pennies, or teach the kids how to read the dates on those coins before swallowing them.

> *If the child shows himself to be incorrigible, he should be decently and quietly beheaded at the age of twelve lest he grow to maturity, marry and perpetuate his kind.*
> —Don Marquis (1878-1937)

Bladder fullness and cardiac ischemia. Can a full bladder trigger an ischemic episode in the myocardium? Have you ever had to urinate so badly that you thought you were going to die? Well, guess what? A recent study has associated a full bladder with triggering ischemic episodes in patients with coronary heart disease. The research, published in the *Journal of the American College of Cardiology* (2000; 36(2): 453-60), studied 40 volunteers with a single, minor atherosclerotic narrowing of a coronary artery. Two catheters were placed in each of the volunteers. One catheter was inserted in a coronary artery to measure blood flow and the other catheter was inserted in the bladder to fill it "to the brim"with water.

With the bladder fully distended, 30 percent of the patients developed chest pain and ECG changes associated with cardiac ischemia. The heart rate increased an average of nine beats per minute and blood flow to the heart decreased by an average of 25 percent.

Whoa, hohohoho!! This study provides fairly convincing evidence that the bladder is connected to the heart. Or at the least it provides fairly convincing evidence that distended bladders can cause ischemia, which may result in heart problems in patients with established coronary artery disease, albeit only mild single vessel disease.

So bladder beware. Heart patients on diuretics should empty their bladders as frequently as possible. Avoid taking long trips without restroom breaks, and time the administration of a diuretic so that a full bladder and a restroom are *not* 250 miles apart!

Henry Ward Beecher, when asked on his deathbed if he could raise his arm, answered, "Well, high enough to hit you, Doctor."

Heart patients and laughter. Patients with heart disease apparently have a lousy sense of humor. When presented with a funny situation, patients with heart disease were 45 percent less likely to laugh than healthy individuals. The lowest risk for heart attack was found among those with the best senses of humor. How do you get a good sense of humor? Well, for one…start hanging around with people who make you laugh. Secondly, rent a few movies that are considered to be funny—if you need a list, give me a call. And third, take yourself less seriously. Learn to laugh at your silly mistakes, laugh when you wear a blue and black sock to work, and don't beat yourself up over every little mishap. Laughter truly is the best medicine. (Michael Miller, MD, Director of Preventive Cardiology, University of Maryland Medical Center, Baltimore)

Zip it when having your blood pressure taken. If there is ever a time to keep your mouth shut, it's while you're having your blood pressure taken. Researchers from the Clinique Cardiologique in Paris found that talking caused a sharp rise in both systolic and diastolic blood pressures in patients with pre-existing hypertension. Moral of the story: Keep your mouth shut when having your blood pressure taken—you'll get a lower reading.

Vacation benefits. Don't skip that annual trip to Aruba or Tibet! Over a nine-year period approximately 13,000 middle-aged men who were healthy but at high risk for coronary artery disease filled out five questionnaires that inquired about their annual vacation habits. After researchers adjusted for their age, education level, and income, frequent vacationers were 29 percent less likely to die from any cause, compared with those who rarely, if ever, vacationed. So, to heck with the daily treadmills—hit the white sandy beaches of the Caribbean for a heart-healthy break from the everyday world of the work-a-holic. And *force* yourself to do it yearly! (*Psychosomatic Medicine,* September/October 2000)

Can mental training improve muscle strength? A new study appears to demonstrate that people can increase muscle power by simply visualizing the exercise. Wow, talk about a mind/body connection. This answers the prayers of every fitness-phobic couch barnacle that has ever existed. The study, led by Guang Yue of the Cleveland Clinic Foundation's Lerner Research Institute, asked if concentration alone might produce physical benefits. Experiments with 30 healthy young adults—who spent 15 minutes daily over 12 weeks imagining using their little finger muscle and their elbow flexor muscles—suggest it may. After 12 weeks of those strenuous mental exercises, little finger strength increased by 35 percent and elbow strength increased by 13.4 percent. The tests involved *no* physical movement of targeted muscles during the "training" period. Does this mean that imaginary exercise can take the place of calorie burning, flexibility and an increase in cardiovascular capacity? Well, not exactly. But, the head researcher, Yue, still contends that imaginary exercises can be hard work. The research involved 50 repetitions per day on a single muscle group. This research may actually hold some promise for individuals with strokes and other neurologic impairments. (Presented at the 2001 annual meeting for the Society for Neuroscience.)

Cancer and the Vatican Radio. It appears as if Vatican Radio may emit enough EMFs (electromagnetic fields) that the neighboring communities are concerned about the higher than normal rates of leukemia associated with long-term exposure to the emissions. Researchers tracked leukemia cases over a 13-year period within a 10-kilometer radius of the transmitters—an area that contains 60,000 people. Typical Italian leukemia figures would have predicted 37 adult deaths, but the study revealed 40. That tiny increase doesn't sound like a huge deal, however a disproportionate share of the 21 cases in men occurred within a 6-km radius of the antennas. Also, all eight cases of leukemia in children, slightly more than expected, occurred within that radius. Leukemia deaths occurred at almost triple the expected rate for men within two kilometers of the 31 antennas and double within the 4-km radius. *(American Journal of Epidemiology,* June 15, 2002*)*

Oya yubi, **the "thumb tribe."** Looks like evolution is changing as a result of video games. Thumbs are becoming as agile as the other four fingers, especially in people under 25 who spend hours every day on Game Boys, cell phones, and other handheld devices. Since the thumbs have become so muscular, they are used for other daily functions, such as ringing a doorbell and even pointing at things. Young people use both thumbs and fingers to push buttons on their cell phones versus the older generation who just use fingers. This is the type of physical change that usually happens over centuries and generations, not just a single generation. (*The WEEK,* April 5, 2002*)*

Does thumb sucking vary with race and color? Yes. Various studies found that 45 percent of American children under the age of four years suck their thumbs compared with 30 percent of Swedish children, 17 percent of Indian children and 1 percent of Eskimo children. Eskimo children usually don't need to suck their thumbs because they are usually carried in their mother's backpacks with a bottle close at hand. Most thumb sucking stops spontaneously by age four.

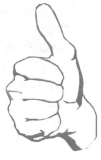

A new use for discarded Barbie dolls. How many Barbie dolls are making their residence in landfills today? Probably too many, so listen up. If you have an old Barbie you would like to discard, call your friendly prosthetic lab before tossing her.

Jennifer Jordan, an engineering student at Duke University Medical Center and her mentor, Jane Bahor, an anaplastologist (one who specializes in producing artificial body parts), have discovered a new use for old, discarded Barbie doll legs. Apparently Barbie's flexible knee joint makes a perfect joint for a flexible prosthetic finger. (Jennifer Jordan, the engineering student, just happened to be in need of a flexible prosthetic finger herself and came up with the idea and presented it to Dr. Bahor.)

The ratchet leg joint mimics a bone, creating a scaffold around which foam is attached and formed into a natural-appearing finger. The joint bends and holds a position, allowing wearers to pick up a pencil, hold a cup, and perform numerous tasks with their new prosthesis. Previous prosthetic fingers were unable to perform the task because they were made with wire and wire doesn't bend and hold the desired position anywhere near what Barbie's leg can do.

Is there any downside to the Barbie-leg-finger prosthesis? Apparently it can be just a bit noisy when the bending occurs. It makes a cracking sound or a clicking noise when put in position.

Can your initials contribute to a longer life span? Men with positive initials, such as VIP (Victor Inman Pearson), or WOW (William Olsen Wyatt), live 4.5 years longer than men whose initials are meaningless (like this study) or considered negative such as BUM (Bruce Ulrich Moore), or SAP (Steven Arthur Perkins). The theory is based on the fact that men with negative initials are teased more as children, which may take its toll in the long run. Back to the "stress" factor. Women with positive initials such as FAB (Frances Anne Parker) lived an average of 3.4 years longer than those with negative initials such as Donna Uma Lund, DUL, or Diana Inez Pearlman, DIP. (Christenfeld N, presentation at the 1997 annual Society of Behavioral Medicine)

If we can't kill you the old fashioned way, like blowing you up, we'll stink you out with an odor bomb. Well, once again, our government has been hard at work spending your hard-earned tax dollars. Experts at the Department of Defense (DOD) have decided that a good way to thwart an enemy attack or squelch a rowdy demonstration would be to release a nasty odor. The DOD gave the Monell Chemical Senses Center in Philadelphia a three-year grant to study the most noxious odors on the face of the planet. The three-year study has been completed and the biological odors found to be the most repugnant were human fecal waste and rotting food. The odor in human fecal matter is from compounds known as skatoles, and rotting foods release rancid-smelling butyric acid and various sulfurous decay by-products. Sooo…the 64-million dollar question is: Do these weapons of mass dispersion work? Apparently an entire building was evacuated due to one of the smells released during the three-year study. And, now we have another secret weapon to stockpile.

Coccyx. Coccyx is from the Greek word *kokkyx*, or "the cuckoo bird." The ancient Greeks gave this name to the rudimentary tail vertebrae of man because of its resemblance to the bill of a cuckoo bird. The coccyx was at one time called "the whistle bone," because of its anatomical relationship to the source of flatus (gas). FYI: The only bone in the body that has absolutely no function is the coccyx, man's vestigial tail.

Speaking of the whistle bone. "If we passed all of the gas we made, everybody would be farting a million times a day," sayeth the guru of gas passing, Dr. Michael Levitt, M.D. and GAS-troenterologist extraordinaire, Director of Research at the Minneapolis Veterans Affairs Medical Center. (By the way, the field of GAS-troenterology is not named after the odiferous emission known as flatus. It is from the Greek word, *gaster,* which means "belly.")

Charley horse is a term commonly used to describe intense pain and stiffness, usually in thigh muscles and especially consequent to athletic stress. The explanation is said to be that Charley was the name given customarily to an elderly, often partially lame horse that was retired from more strenuous service and reserved for family use. When stretching in the morning in bed, bend the toes backward (not forward) in order to prevent a charley horse from the stretch. (Source: personal experience.)

I love my job—things could be a lot worse. When you have a bad day at the office try this for therapy. On your way home from work, stop at your pharmacy and purchase a rectal thermometer made by Johnson and Johnson. When you get home change to very comfortable clothing and lie down on your bed. Open the package and remove the thermometer. Carefully place it on the bedside table so that it will not become chipped or broken. Take out the material that comes with the thermometer and read it. You will notice that in small print there is a statement, "Every rectal thermometer made by Johnson and Johnson is personally tested." Now close your eyes and repeat out loud, "I am so glad I do not work for quality control at the Johnson and Johnson Company." Always remember that someone has a job worse than yours.

Whispering endearments. If you're going to whisper sweet nothings in your beloved's ear, make sure you do it in their left ear if you want them to remember it. Scientists in Huntsville, Texas, report a 64 percent recall rate when emotional words are spoken into the left ear compared to a 58 percent recall in the right ear. This greater recall is because the right hemisphere of the brain processes emotional stimuli and it controls the left ear. (*Men's Health,* October 2001)

Wrinkles and driving. If you spend inordinate amounts of time behind the wheel, you may just be wrinkled on the left side of your face much more than the right side due to the sun beating down on your face through the car window. To be on the safe side you might want to apply sunscreen to the left side of your face before a long haul.

Sex and wrinkles. Clinical neuropsychologist David Weeks of the Royal Edinburgh Hospital, questioned 3,500 people who had been judged to look young for their age. Apparently the one common denominator amongst the group was the number of times they had sex per week. Having sex three times a week appeared to take seven to twelve years off their looks. What they *didn't* find is that having sex *more* than three times per week reduces our age even further. And, casual sex, by the way, seems to increase the aging process because it increases stress levels.

> *Reality is the leading cause of stress amongst those in touch with it.*
> —Lily Tomlin

Chapter 2

The Scoop, the Score & Numbers Galore

> **The Ultimate Generalist**
> *He who learns less and less about more and more until he can tell you almost nothing about everything.*

Abdominal fat. A study of 4,769 male runners under age 50 found that even dedicated athletes fight an uphill battle with weight gain as they age. Per decade, an average 6-foot male will add 0.75 inches, or 3.3 pounds of flab to his waist. (*Scientific American*, July 1977)

Age. In 1900 the average life span was only 48 years for men and 46 years for women. Only 4 percent of the U.S. population was over 65. Today, American men can expect to live to the age of 74 and women to 80. About 4.2 million Americans are 85 and older, and over 100,000 have reached their 100th birthday. Researchers from the Cambridge University and Germany's Max Planck Institute for Demographic Research have calculated that ever since 1840, people born in any given year have generally lived three months longer than those born the previous year.

Just how long can we live? Living to be the ripe old age of 100 is an increasing possibility for thousands of Americans. This fact, not lost on the Hallmark greeting card company, has prompted the release of 70,000 "Happy 100th Birthday" cards for this year. Centenarians are the most rapidly growing segment of the population. The prediction of one million centenarians in America by the year 2050 is not too far-fetched. And, there I'll sit—rocking on the porch of the nursing home and celebrating the *big* one-oh-oh.

So, if you're going to live that long, are you aging too fast? Here are a couple of fun tests you can do to assess your functional age, not your actual age. Actual age just means how many years you have been on this earth, functional age means how well you're coping with being on this earth for all of those years.

1) Pinch the skin on the back of your hand for five seconds and time how long it takes to flatten out completely. If you are less than 50, the skin should return to normal within 5 seconds; by age 60 it will take 10 to15 seconds, and by age 70 the typical time is 35 to 55 seconds. This measures the degree of deterioration of the connective tissue under the skin.

2) How long can you stand on one leg with your eyes closed before falling flat on your face? Take your shoes off or wear tennis shoes for this test. Stand on a hard surface (sans rug) with both feet together, and close your eyes. If you're right handed, lift your left foot six inches off the ground, bending your knee at a 45° angle. Have a friend close by to catch you just in case you decide to take a nosedive. Perform the test three times and calculate the average time. On average, a 100 percent decline occurs from 20 to 80 years of age. Most 20-year-olds are able to stand 30 seconds or more whereas most 80-year-olds are unable to hold the pose longer than a few seconds. Where did you "fall" in that group?

Live a Little, Laugh a Lot

Aging and ear lobe growth. A British study has quantified one of the dreaded complications of aging—the elongation of the ear lobe. As men age, their ears grow an average of .008 inches per year. This is the equivalent of more than one-third of an inch over a 50-year life span. Add another 40 years to that life span and another third of an inch and those ear lobes may just be tickling the tops of your shoulders.

Aging and "long in the tooth." This is a slang term for getting older, but what does it mean in the literal sense of the word? Two mechanisms are responsible for older people growing long in the tooth. First of all, bone mineral content is lost with aging due to osteoporosis and periodontal disease, and the maxilla and mandible are not exceptions to this rule. This loss causes the gum tissue to retract from the teeth. In addition, our gums tend to shrink with age and this also contributes to the appearance of being long in the tooth.

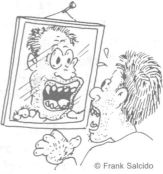
© Frank Salcido

Age and sex frequency. If you are 18 to 29 years of age the average number of times you have sex per year is 81; 30 to 39 years of age, the average number is 80 times per year; 40 to 49, 65 times per year; 50 to 59, 46 times per year; 60 to 69, 27 times per year, and 70 or older, 9 times per year.

Airbags. Lab studies have shown that air bag deployment can result in peak acoustic pressure of 170 decibels (a pig squeals at 108 decibels, a chain saw is 103 decibels and your husband's snoring can be as loud as 80 decibels). A 170-decibel pressure can cause acute pain and long-term significant hearing loss. (Morris MS, Borja LP. Air bag deployment and hearing loss. *Arch Otolaryngol Head Neck Surg* 1998:124(5):507)

Airplane etiquette. Thirty-two percent of women and 24 percent of men refuse to fall asleep on airplanes because they are afraid they will start drooling.

Babies cry an average of 4,000 times before reaching the age of two. (Lutz T. *Crying: The Natural and Cultural History of Tears*. 1999. Norton)

Bad breath. The salivary glands produce between 500 to 1,500 ml of saliva per day. During waking hours this saliva washes over the teeth and tongue and helps to rid the mouth of bacterial and food particles upon which bacteria feast. Bad breath develops during sleep when saliva production slows to just less than 10 ml at night. The mouth becomes a stagnant reservoir of 1,600 billion bacteria feeding on dead buccal (cheek) cells and the remaining meal from dinner (especially if you don't floss before bedtime).

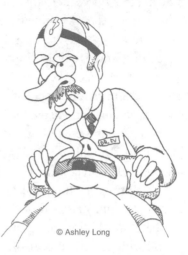

© Ashley Long

The bacteria break down the cells and food particles into sulfur compounds imparting that early morning "boiled egg" breath. The cure— floss before bedtime and brush your teeth and your tongue.

Note: Hormonal fluctuations also contribute to good or bad breath. Women have more of a problem with bad breath during ovulation. The increase in estrogen during this time causes the blood vessels in the gums surrounding each tooth to contract, forming a crevice that allows fluid to pool, attracting bacteria.

Body numbers—fascinating facts:

- Each individual is so unique, that the odds against duplication by the same parents are about 144 billion to 1.

- Six pounds of skin cover 20 square feet of surface on the average adult. Sitting perfectly still you will shed more than a million flakes of skin every hour. Estimates indicate that there are approximately 650,000 microorganisms per square inch of human skin. In fact, there are more of these microorganisms on each of us than there are people in this world.

- The eyelid has the thinnest skin. It is less than 1/500th of an inch thick.

- The average adult has between 40 and 50 billion fat cells.

- The body has approximately 20 feet of small intestine and 6 feet of large intestine, with a surface area of more than 100 feet, or five times the area of the body's skin. The intestines process 40 tons of food over the course of 70 years. The intestines process food at about an inch per minute.

- The average person will take one billion steps in life and walk about 77,000 miles, landing on the 26 bones of each foot with a force triple his/her body weight.

- A man's testicles produce more sperm per second (approximately 2,000) than a woman's ovaries produce mature eggs (approximately 430) in a reproductive lifetime.

- The female egg (ovum or oocyte) is the largest cell in the human body. It is about 1/180 of an inch in diameter. Interestingly, the sperm is the smallest cell in the human body. And we wonder who's the dominant sex? It takes about 175,000 sperm to weigh as much as a single egg.

- Eight million red blood cells are produced in the bone marrow every second. At any given moment we have 25 trillion red blood cells, 35 billion white blood cells, and 1.5 trillion platelets circulating through our blood vessels.

- The human brain has 100 billion neurons. How big is 100 billion? An appropriate analogy would be the Amazon rain forest. It stretches for 2,700,000 square miles and it contains about 100 billion trees. To consider the number of connections between the 100 billion neurons, consider the number of leaves on the trees of the Amazon rain forest.

- The 3-pound brain stores 100 trillion bits of information over the course of 70 years, equal to 500,000 sets of the *Encyclopedia Britannica*, which, when stacked, would reach 442 miles. Approximately 100,000 chemical reactions occur in the brain every second. Forty-five miles of nerves send impulses as rapidly as 325 miles per hour. The human hand has 1,300 nerve endings per square inch.

- Is there life after death? Who knows? However, we do know that there is brain wave activity after death. Cortical activity can occur for an average of 37 hours. The longest brain activity recorded after death was 168 hours or right about seven days.

- Each hair follicle on the head is capable of producing 30 feet of hair in a lifetime. Approximately 125,000 hairs (range is 120,000 hairs to 150,000 hairs) grow in the scalp, with about 45 hairs lost each day. Uncut over a lifetime, a head of hair could theoretically reach a length of 30 feet. The current record is 16 feet 11 inches and it belongs to Hoo Sateow of Thailand. (*Guinness Book of World Records*, 2003)

- Every day we pump 21,000 gallons of blood through 62,000 miles of blood vessels. Over a lifetime, a normal human heart will pump enough blood to fill 13 supertankers, each with a capacity of one million barrels. The heart does enough work each day to lift the body one mile straight up in the air. The heart pumps blood out of the left ventricle into the aorta to be distributed throughout the vascular system. The pressure in the aorta is such that if the aorta were opened, blood would spout a column six feet high.

- Let's talk about heartbeats for a minute. Some researchers have theorized that each of us is pre-programmed to have only a certain number of heartbeats per lifetime. Which means of course, that the faster you use them up, like with running, the quicker you will use up your allotment. (How's this for a perfect reason *not* to exercise?)

Word Origin

Aorta may have originated from the Greek noun, *aorter*, which meant "a strap over the shoulder to hang anything on." When observing the thoracic and abdominal cavities of a cadaver, the aorta looks like a sturdy strap from which all of the internal organs "hang," including the heart, kidneys, and abdominal organs.

The artery (Greek for "windpipe") was originally named by the Greek physician Praxagoras who thought that the arteries carried only air. Of course, he studied corpses and the arteries of corpses tend to be empty, so he was partially correct.

- Well, don't toss those running shoes so fast. An exercise physiologist, who most likely was also a trivia buff, whipped out his calculator one day, did some fancy figuring and reported the following results: The average non-marathon running human has a resting heart rate of 72 beats per minute, and an average life span of 75 years. This works out to 2.832 billion beats per lifetime. In comparison, the average 20- to 60-year-old conditioned runner who averages 45 minutes of jogging per day, four to five times per week, has a resting heart rate of 55 per minute. His exercise-induced heart rate is 180 beats per minute. Calculations show that he would run out of heartbeats by the age of 94, almost 20 years after his non-exercising counterpart.

> *The only reason I would take up jogging is so that I could hear heavy breathing again.*
> —Erma Bombeck

- The heart beats faster when you're arguing if and when to have sex than it does during the actual sex act itself.

- The human heart beats about 100,000 times in a 24-hour period. It takes approximately 20 seconds for a drop of blood to make it though the entire circulatory system.

- We breathe one pint of air 17 times per minute, inhaling 11,000 liters of air in one day and taking in 78 million gallons of air in an average life span. This amount of air is enough to fill the Hindenburg (the doomed dirigible), one and a half times. A man snoozing in a hammock may absorb only ½ pint of oxygen per minute; however, a runner trying to break the world's record in the mile, may suck up more than five quarts of oxygen in that same minute.

- There are approximately 2.5 million nephrons to do the dirty work of excreting our metabolic waste products via both kidneys. Nephrons are composed of a filtering apparatus (called the glomerulus), and tubules. The average 25-year-old filters 180 liters of urine filtrate per day. Tubules do the lion's share of reabsorption and fine tuning the urine filtrate. Of the 180 liters filtered, 178 liters are reabsorbed by the renal tubules. If the tubules of all 2.5 million nephrons were stretched out, they would stretch for approximately 50 miles, or 80 kilometers.

- Under normal circumstances the average American adult passes between 200 to 2,000 ml of gas per 24 hours with a mean of 600 ml. The average number of times an average American adult passes gas is 13.6 +/- 6 per 24 hours. The basal flatal rate (or BFR as acronyms go) averages 15 ml per hour but substantially increases after one ingests a meal, any meal. For example, following your basic breakfast, one notes an increase in the number of times gas is passed and the amount passed. This rate is referred to as the PPFR or the postprandial flatal rate. The average amount passed after a meal is 100 ml per expulsion. You can only imagine the lunch crowd riding the elevator to the 110th floor of the Sears Tower together. What about gas-producing foods such as baked beans? This brings to mind the age-old question, "Why don't we serve baked beans at indoor functions?" They are always served at outdoor picnics, kind of a fall and spring-time food. A meal with baked beans included increases the PPFR to a walloping 176 ml per hour.

- The everyday sit-up done the wrong way (the way you learned back in high school) burdens the lumbar vertebrae with as much pressure as deep-sea divers feel at 570 feet. A high jump may load the femur with approximately 20,000 pounds of stress upon landing.

An Alaskan Eskimo father freed his son's tongue that was frozen to a handrail by urinating on it. As a general rule, running warm water over a tongue frozen to a handrail would suffice, but access to warm, running water was limited in this particular situation. (Letter—N Engl J Med)

- The human as a light bulb—the resting human gives off as much heat as a 150-watt light bulb. How about the amount of heat a woman gives off during a hot flash? It's got to be ten times that amount.

- The interaction of light with pigments in the retina, the process that allows vision, takes about 200 femtoseconds. What is a femtosecond? It is a millionth of a billionth of a second. As we all know, light travels from the object we're looking at to the eye and through the optic nerve and optic radiations to the occipital cortex for interpretation. Until about 400 years ago, it was believed that there was a "force" that exited from the eye to see the object.

- If it were possible to drain all of the water from a 72.6 kg (160-pound) man, his dehydrated body would weigh a mere 29 kg or 64 pounds. Of that 64 pounds, 19 would be bone.

- Our bones have two types of strength—tensile strength (the resistance to being pulled apart) and compressive strength (the resistance to being compressed or crumbled).On average, the adult bone has tensile strength of 12,000 to 17,000 pounds per square inch and a compressive strength of approximately 18,000 to 25,000 pounds per square inch. Let's compare this to the mighty white oak tree shall we? The tensile strength of the white oak tree along the grain is only 12,500 pounds per square inch whereas the compressive strength of the white oak along the grain is only 7,000 pounds per square inch.

- Fingernails grow at a rate of approximately 1 cm every three months. Nail growth is faster on the right hand, on the larger fingers, during daylight and in summer. Minor nail trauma and nail biting may enhance nail growth, while illness usually slows it down.

- The outer layer of skin, the epidermis, replaces itself every four weeks.

- Well, here's an anthropological gem that will keep you up at night. Our teeth are getting smaller. Yes, and we can blame this fascinating fact on the fact that we are cooking our food instead of just ripping it off the bone or yanking it directly off the plant and chewing on it for long periods of time. Teeth have shrunk in size by about 50 percent over the past 100,000 years. Don't worry; you won't wake up tomorrow completely toothless. Teeth are shrinking, but only at a rate of 1 percent per 1,000 years.

- The bad news: Each minute of our lives 300 million cells die. The good news: We replace lost cells as fast as they die. The final news: If we didn't replace the cells we would be dead in 230 days.

- It has been estimated that approximately 35 billion cells divide each day in a healthy adult, and any of these divisions could produce a rogue cell population that continues to grow without constraint. Uncontrolled cell growth is called cancer. We make about 100 cancer cells per day but fortunately our immune system recognizes these cancer cells as foreign and immediately destroys the cells before they have the chance to develop into a malignant tumor.

- The sinuses produce a pint to a quart of mucus every day.

- The average number of dreams per year is 1,460, or about 4 per night. We spend two of every twenty-four hours dreaming, adding up to more than five years of our lives. Approximately 12 percent of male dreams have sexual content. This is certainly contrary to the popular belief that sex is the *only* thing men dream about. Most of us dream in color, not black and white. It may take days to transfer memories from the short-term memory area to the long-term memory bank. The dreaming brain may shift information back and forth between the two areas for as long as a week before it finally settles into long-term memory. So, if you learn an important concept for a test on Monday but the test isn't until Thursday, be sure to get three solid nights of good sleep so that the concept will "stick." Are you a lucid dreamer? Lucid dreamers are aware of their dreams and can actually change the dream any way they wish. Lucid dreamers can change the participants, the circumstances and even the outcome to their advantage.

- The ability to taste diminishes with age. If you place a small electrical stimulus with a metallic taste on the tongue, 82 percent of the 20- to 30-year-olds will perceive it, whereas only 16 over the age of 52 will recognize the taste.

- It takes 17 muscles to give you a great big smile and 43 muscles to give you a great big frown. In terms of energy expenditure it would appear that smiling would be the most energy efficient. However, in terms of caloric expenditure it would appear that frowning would be your best bet. So, if weight loss is your goal and you're counting calories, start frowning. Let's move to the side of the head for a second. There are actually 6 muscles in the human ear. Can you think of any logical reason as to why you might have six muscles in your ear? This harkens back to our distant past when our ancestors were able to "cock" their ears in order to listen for deadly predators. Today the ability to cock one's ears simply serves as a party pleaser when the conversation lulls.

- The duration of a typical yawn is six seconds. If you think about yawning, you will most likely yawn. Even blind individuals, when hearing a tape of a yawn, will yawn. Did you just yawn?

Animals and insects vs. humans. In this era that places so much emphasis on athletic prowess, we tend to forget that our athletic records are rather paltry compared to our furry and feathery friends.

- The human world record for the long jump is barely over 29 feet. However, the Australian kangaroo can jump 42 feet without breaking a sweat. The human high jump record measures out around 7 feet 11 inches, however, the kangaroo once again has us beat. He can leap10 feet in a single bound.

- The human record for cruising through the water using the crawl stroke is about 5.3 miles per hour. Don't even think about swimming away from a hungry crocodile. The crocodile cruises at 20 miles per hour in the swamp. A penguin will blow past you at 22 miles per hour and never look back. The sailfish and the swordfish swim more than 60 miles per hour. (Even if you make it to shore and start running full throttle, the crocodile can catch up to you. The croc has been clocked at 30 miles per hour on land.)

- Heck, we can't even *fall* through the air with the greatest of speed. A free-falling human skydiver can reach 185 miles per hour, but he will be promptly passed by the peregrine falcon plunging at speeds up to 275 miles per hour. The longest recorded flight of a chicken is 13 seconds—and that's 13 seconds longer than any human can fly.

- A fly has a lightning flash reflex and reaction time of less than one two hundredth of a second—ten times quicker than that of a fly swatter attached to the human hand.

- If all of the gyri (ridges) of the cerebral cortex were flattened out our brain would cover over two square feet. In contrast, if all of the ridges of the rat's cortex were flattened out, the brain would cover an area the size of a postage stamp. Let's move up a notch on the evolutionary totem pole. If all of the ridges of the chimpanzee cortex were flattened out, the brain would cover an area the size of a piece of standard typing paper.

- The night owl (great-horned owl) has 14 vertebrae in its neck, giving it the unique ability to swirl its head through three-fourths (about 270°) of a complete circle. It needs this mobility because of the size of its eyes, which are so large that there is no room in the head for the extraocular muscles that move the eyes from side to side or up and down.

- A 10-gram hummingbird burns ten times as much oxygen per gram of body weight as an energetic, exercising human. To do this, a hummingbird's heart beats about 1,440 times per minute. The heart of an exercising human pounds anywhere from 110 to 220 beats per minute.

- A giraffe has the same number of cervical vertebrae in his/her neck as a human—and that would be seven. However, the *size* of the vertebrae is the major difference in the length of the human neck as compared to the giraffe neck.

- An elephant's brain is five and a half times bigger than a human brain. It weighs about 17 pounds as compared to the 3-pound human brain. Compared to body size, however, the elephant's brain is only 0.2 percent of its total body weight as compared to the human brain, which is 2.33 percent of body weight. The elephant's trunk has 100,000 muscles controlling its movements.

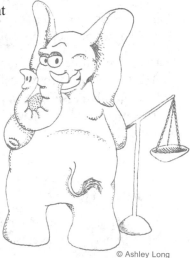

- An elephant's heart weighs 28.5 pounds. An elephant's testicle weighs 5.5 pounds and an elephant's penis is three to four feet long. The human penis is 1.5 inches to 19 inches. The combined average weight of a Chinese man's testicles is 19.01

© Ashley Long

Live a Little, Laugh a Lot

grams. The average combined weight of a Danish man's testicles is 42 grams.

- Sheep produce a magnanimous amount of methane gas. The 70 million sheep living in New Zealand release 2.5 billion gallons of methane into the earth's atmosphere every week. A geophysicist from the New Zealand Institute of Nuclear Science believes that this methane might be a major contributor to global warming. This same researcher, obviously with time on his hands and a calculator nearby, noted that if you hooked up a sheep to the carburetor of a car, you could run it for several kilometers per day. To power the same vehicle by people, you would need an entire football team and a couple of kegs of beer.

- The olfactory bulbs, that part of the bloodhound's nose that performs the task of smelling, is 50 times larger and one million times more sensitive than a human nose. Sue, the most famous dinosaur residing at the Museum of Natural History in Chicago, had olfactory bulbs the size of grapefruits. The sense of olfaction was obviously important in the dinosaur age since the majority of Sue's cranial vault was consumed by her two olfactory bulbs. As a comparison, the human olfactory bulb is about the size of a match head.

- The tongue of the giant anteater of South America is 22 to 24 inches long. It slurps up about 25,000 ants per day. The human tongue can't even compete with that of the giant anteater. Stick yours out right now and measure it.

- The healthy human liver weighs approximately three pounds, or 2 percent of a 160-pound (72 kg) male. The great white shark, on the other hand, weighing in at 800 pounds, has a liver weighing 20 percent of his total body weight or 160 pounds. Why would a shark's liver comprise 20 percent of the body's weight? The shark must subsist for weeks and sometimes months on its fat reserves, and the liver just so happens to be where the shark stores fat.

The belly button (also known as the umbilicus). Thirty-eight percent of the American population will clean their belly button every day. Speaking of belly buttons—One day, while having his abdomen examined, a young boy asked the examiner if she had ever "stuck her finger in her belly button and 'smelt' it." The examiner was somewhat taken aback by this blunt question, and of course, she had to think about it for a moment. "Of course not," she replied, rather indignantly. The young boy, unfazed by her indignation, proceeded to tell her that if she stuck her finger in her belly button and 'smelt' it, it would smell "just like butt!" After the exam she continued to be intrigued by the question and decided to ask an expert on the relationship between smelly belly buttons and smelly butts. Apparently there *is* a connection and that connection has its origins in the developing embryo. The umbilicus (belly button) is a remnant of the GI tract in the fetus. When the GI tract is colonized with normal bacteria approximately three months after birth, it also colonizes the belly button. Hence, the belly button *does* smell like butt. And, your homework assignment for tonight is… (and you have to dig deep).

Belly buttons and lint—The *Ig Nobel* prizes for the silly side of science. Every year awards are presented by the Cambridge-based magazine *The Annals of Improbable Research* or *AIR*. These awards honor those whose work "cannot or should not be reproduced" in the world of scientific research. The 2002 winner in interdisciplinary research was Karl Kruszelinski of Australia (University of Sydney). He conducted an exhaustive study on bellybutton lint sent in by 4,799 volunteers. His conclusion: "The typical generator of bellybutton lint or fluff is a slightly overweight, middle-aged male with a hairy abdomen." (*Ig Nobels*, October 2002)

Diabetes update. The numbers keep increasing. A whopping increase of 165 percent in newly diagnosed Type 2 diabetes is expected by the year 2050. Among ethnic groups, the biggest increase is expected to be among black men (363 percent), with black women expected to see the second highest increase (217 percent). The study, reported in the November issue of *Diabetes Care*, projects that the highest increase in prevalence will be in the over 75 age group. "Why, why, why?" you ask.

Three reasons come to mind in a jiffy. Lifestyle changes related to obesity (sedentary lifestyle and fast food fanaticism), the aging population, and the changing racial composition have all been proposed as reasons.

Jiffy. I'll be back in a jiffy. A jiffy, for your information, is an actual unit of time in the world of computer science. It is one one-hundredth of a second. You can't even *go away* in a jiffy, so how in the heck can you be back in one?

Heart attacks. Only 50 percent of the patients who have had a heart attack (myocardial infarction) have serum cholesterol levels above 240 mg/dL prior to the episode. Obviously serum cholesterol must not be the only reason for heart attacks then, eh? And that's where the "inflammation" theory enters into the fray. A new blood test called the C-reactive protein measures the amount of inflammation in the arteries and may be used in the future as frequently as cholesterol levels to monitor heart disease risk.

Hip fractures in women. The risk of hip fracture at age 45 is 0.3 per 1,000; the risk of hip fracture at age 85 is 20 per 1,000. The lifetime risk of sustaining any osteoporetic fracture (hip, vertebrae, or wrist) is 50 percent compared to only 9 percent for breast cancer and 31 percent for coronary artery disease.

Of 100 older persons (older than age 70) with a hip fracture:
- 30 will recover to pre-fracture functional status within one year
- 30 will die before the year is over
- 40 will survive but only partially recover; of the 40, 20 will require some assistance with activities of daily living and the other 20 will never make it out of the nursing home or assisted living facility.

There is a 50 to 60 percent lower risk of hip fractures in women who have taken estrogen replacement therapy (ERT) for six years. ERT delays bone loss but it doesn't prevent it altogether. A woman who has been on ERT for 20 years has a bone density of a woman who is 10 years younger. Even with ERT there is a very gradual age-dependent bone loss.

There are 25 million women with a risk of hip fracture in the U.S. today. The risk is equal to the combined risk of breast cancer, ovarian cancer, and uterine cancer.

Jog backwards. Try jogging backwards when you are out taking your daily walk or run. Jogging backward burns 32 percent more calories than jogging forward. The feet touch the ground for shorter periods of time while jogging backward, so leg muscles must work harder and move faster.

Life and death. Every hour, 15,020 people are born throughout the world. In that same hour, 6,279 people die.

Maternal mortality. Maternal mortality has been an under recognized issue worldwide despite an estimated 600,000 maternal deaths per year. Put in numerical perspective, this is the equivalent to six jumbo jet crashes per day with the deaths of all 250 passengers on board, all of them in the reproductive years of life. There is also marked inequity in geographic distribution since 95 percent of the deaths occur in developing countries.

Risky business. Everything you do in your life is risky, including sleep. In fact, one out of every two million Americans (130 individuals to be exact) will die every year when they fall out of bed during sleep.

If you don't die from falling out of bed, you can be injured while lying in bed. That is, 1 in 400 will sustain an injury, usually from some sort of structural failure, such as a headboard collapsing on the head sleeping adjacent to it, or the frame deciding to give way under all of that accumulated weight gained over the years.

Of course, what you're doing in that bed may also contribute to your risk of injury or dying. It appears as if middle-aged men (considered to be 35 and over in this instance), have the highest risk of dying in bed whilst in the throes of passion with someone *other* than their usual partner, the middle-aged wife. The exact risk is less than 1 percent.

An FYI: Most heart attacks that occur during sexual intercourse happen when men are cheating on their wives. Dr. Graham Jackson of St. Thomas' Hospital in London actually did a study that found that 75 percent of the cases of sudden death during sexual activity involved people who were taking part in an extramarital affair. The typical maximal heart rate attained during sexual intercourse is about 100 beats per minute with your usual partner—certainly not a high enough rate to put any extra workload on the heart. In fact, it takes about the same amount of energy to climb the stairs to the bedroom as it does to do "the business" with your usual partner. When making love to a mistress or any other non-routine partner, a man's heart rate increases to an average of 130 per minute. Flings with a younger woman are especially dangerous because the older male partner struggles to keep up with the sexual demands of that "frisky young thang." (Berry E, Conti CR. Post MI care: Guidelines and rationales you can use. *Internal Medicine* 1999; 20(8): 7; *London Daily News,* December 20, 2002)

If you make it through the night without any of the above catastrophic events, there is a 1 in 350 chance of being electrocuted while turning off the alarm clock or turning on the bedside lamp. Once the feet hit the floor running, there is a 1 in 20,000 chance of falling and sustaining a fatal head injury.

Now that you have made it safely into the bathroom, the perils of the porcelain bowl await the unsuspecting male. According to D. Borg's *Book of Risks* (2001), 1 in 6,500 Americans are injured every year using the toilet. The nature of the injury can only be surmised from the information provided—98 percent of the injured are of the male persuasion, hence it doesn't take a doctorate in reproductive anatomy to deduce the most likely appendage injured via the toilet bowl seat.

> ## Case study
> *A 412-pound woman fell head first out of bed, knocked herself unconscious, and was suffocated by her own bosom. "Her enormous breasts had fallen down over her face in such a way that she couldn't get air through her nose or mouth" a police officer said. The 47-year-old woman was said to have worn a 52EEE bra.* Ouch

Now it's time for the shower. The average American faces barely a one in a million chance of being seriously injured in the shower, unless one decides to shave in the shower, increasing the risk of injury to 1 in 7,000.

It's now time to get ready for work. Dressing for work poses special hazards. An individual faces a 1 in 2,600 annual risk of being injured by a zipper, a snap, or some other fastener. This obviously makes Velcro much more appealing as we age and our manual dexterity declines. And of course, with the zipper injuries as well as the toilet seat covers, that gender "thing" comes to mind.

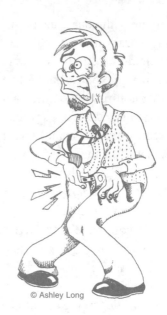
© Ashley Long

It's 7:30 a.m. and time for work. The odds of being killed while walking to work are 1 in 40,000; however, it is still safer to walk to work than to hop in the car. The risk increases to 1 in 11,000 once you're in the car. If you are a pedestrian, your risk of dying in a motor vehicle accident is 1 in 40,000. Your combined risk of dying in a motor vehicle accident, whether as a passenger, pedestrian or driver, is 1 in 5,600.

Once you have arrived at work, the odds of dying at work are directly related to the type of job you do. If you are an office worker, your annual likelihood of dying in a job-related accident is 1 in 37,000...unless, of course, your office has the word *POST* in front of it. Then the odds increase considerably.

While you're at work, what is the risk of having something stolen from your house, car or even your purse while you're away from your desk? The odds of having property stolen in a lifetime are 1 in 14. The odds of being the victim of a violent crime in a lifetime are 1 in 31. And, you have a 1 in 11,000 chance that the violent crime will be a homicide. Here's a "surprise"—the most likely weapon used to commit homicide is a gun. Now that's a big duh. The most likely month to commit a homicide is the hot, sweltering month of August. The least likely month for a homicide is February. The most likely day to commit a homicide is New Year's Day.

Risky business—another way to look at it. John Paling, a former biology professor at the University of Oxford, came up with what he describes as a Richter scale to gauge the dangers of daily living. He came up with the idea after observing a woman smoking a cigarette while inquiring about the benefits of buying a water-purification kit.

If I had to live my past life over again I'd make all the same mistakes—only sooner.
—Tallulah Bankhead

He describes these risks with a range from one in one trillion to one in one. He also gives negative and positive numbers for these risks, so for example a one in one trillion would be a negative six risk versus a one in one risk which would be a positive six risk. The midpoint, or zero on the scale represents a one in a million risk. Paling describes the negative two to negative four risk on this scale as one-in-a-kind risks, the chance of something happening once a year in the entire U.S. He also describes this as the "Bobbitt zone," which we all know would be the chance of a penis being chopped off by a unhappy wife. So then, here are a few examples on Paling's so-called Richter scale of risks:

- One in 1 million to 1 in 10 million risk of dying from a lightning strike

- One in 1 million to 1 in 10 million risk of dying from cancer by eating a charbroiled steak once a week

- One in 1 million is the point below which the FDA deems any risk of cancer from a food additive too small to be of concern over a lifetime

- One in 1 million risk of a woman being killed by a husband or lover

- One in 1 million chance of drowning in a bathtub

- One in 1 in 100,000 extra risk of cancer from cosmic rays for a Denver resident compared with someone living in New York City

- One in 100,000 extra risk of cancer from eating a peanut butter sandwich every day

- One in 10,000 to 1 in 100,000 risk of cancer from drinking one 'lite' beer a day

- One in 10,000 risk of becoming a murder victim

- One in 10,000 risk of dying in childbirth

- One in 10,000 risk of dying from driving a motor vehicle

- One in 1,000 to 1in 10,000 risk of arriving in the emergency room for a treatment for an injury from a sink or toilet

- One in 100 to 1 in 1,000 risk for dying from some form of cancer
    (*Up to Your Armpits in Alligators? How to Sort Out What Risks Are Worth Worrying About.* John and Sean Paling, January 1997)

Roller coaster rides and head injuries. The G-forces generated by the newest, highest, and fastest roller coasters exceed those experienced by space-shuttle astronauts and may be the number one cause for the increased incidence of head, neck, back and brain injuries as well as fatalities observed in the 1990s. The risk is 1 in 124,000 but this risk seriously underestimates the risk because it doesn't include the major amusement parks referred to as "fixed-site" parks, such as Disney World, Six Flags, Universal Studios, and the other big ones. These injuries can occur in young, old, male, female—so anyone complaining of neurological symptoms, especially in the summer months, should be asked if they have been on any roller coaster rides lately. (*Annals of Emergency Medicine* 2002; 39(1):65)

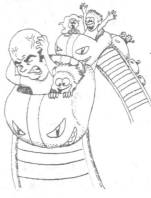

© Ashley Long

Sex. Every 24 hours there are 100 million acts of sexual intercourse around the world. This results in 910,000 conceptions and 350,000 cases of sexually transmitted disease per day. Americans have the most lifetime sex partners, 14.3 compared to the Chinese who average only 2.1. (*World Health Organization,* June, 2001)

Sigmund Freud. Freud's fee for one hour of psychoanalysis in 1895 was $25.00. Adjusted for inflation today, that fee would be $160.

Q: How many Freudians does it take to change a light bulb?

A. Six. Five to change the bulb and one to hold the penis.

Smoking. Two studies in the April 1996 issue of *Pediatrics* quantitate the problems children face from secondhand smoke in the household environment. The following is a summary of the findings:

- Mothers who smoke during pregnancy have a 50 percent higher chance of having a mentally-retarded child than those who do not smoke. The risk increases to 75 percent for mothers who smoke a pack or more a day.

- Secondhand smoke is linked to between 354,000 and 2.2 million middle-ear infections per year.

- Secondhand smoke doubles the chance that a child's tonsils will have to be removed.

- Household smoking results in 307,000 to 522,000 cases of asthma in kids under 15 and results in 529,000 trips to the pediatrician.

- Between 250,000 and 436,000 cases of bronchitis and 115,000 to 190,000 cases of pneumonia in children under five years of age are the result of secondhand smoke.

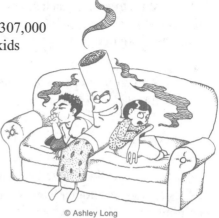

© Ashley Long

- Between 284 and 360 children die per year as a result of secondhand smoke.

- Secondhand smoke might just lower your child's IQ. In a recent study from Cincinnati Children's Hospital Medical Center (October 2002), children with the highest level of cotinine, a by-product of nicotine, had the worst scores on intelligence tests. Just one parent smoking was enough to lower the IQ by two points.

- Women who smoke 15 or more cigarettes per day are twice as likely to have a colicky baby than mothers who don't smoke.

Smoking and the heart. Smoking just one to three cigarettes a day can cause just as much damage to heart vessels as smoking a pack of cigarettes a day. (JA Ambrose, M.D., St. Vincent Catholic Medical Centers, New York, July 2002)

Smoking cigars and the heart. Smoking just one cigar per day increases the risk of death from coronary artery disease by 30 percent in men aged 75 and younger.

Smoking Kents in the '50s. If you smoked the cigarette brand, Kents, in the 1950s, your risk of an asbestos-related cancer known as mesothelioma is substantially increased—even if you gave up smoking years and years ago. It appears as if this particular brand of cigarettes contained crocidolite, a type of asbestos that is considered to be the most carcinogenic of all. Each puff from one Kent carried more than 131 asbestos structures (each structure contained hundreds of crocidolite fibers). Just for the record—11.7 *billion* Kent cigarettes were sold though May of 1956. (*Journal of Cancer Research,* June 1, 1997)

Smoking gun. Every two weeks approximately 15,385 people die of smoking-related diseases in the U.S.

Sneezing. One 11-year-old girl was admitted to the University of New Mexico Hospital after sneezing 20 times per minute for three weeks. Another 17-year-old female had a history of continuous sneezing for 154 days. And yet another woman sneezed for three years at a rate of 25 per minute.

Why do we sneeze? It was once thought that a healthy sneeze served to cleanse the brain. Hippocrates, with all of his infinite wisdom, considered the sneeze as a dangerous sign of lung disease, but that it was curative for hiccups. Hmmm—even Hippocrates was wrong on occasion.

Approximately 20 percent of the population sneeze when they walk out into the sunlight or when they look at a bright light. This is known as the photic sneeze reflex and has been described in the literature for centuries—actually as far back as Hippocrates. The exact physiologic mechanism for this effect is unknown, however, it is believed to be due to intricate connections in the visual pathways that activate the receptors in the upper respiratory system.

Research suggests that the photic sneeze is an inherited trait and is passed to the offspring in an autosomal dominant pattern. In other words, if one of your parents has the photic sneeze, your chance of inheriting the photic sneeze is 50:50. There is even a clever acronym to describe this reflex—*ACHOO*—**a**utosomal dominant **c**ompelling **h**elio-**o**pthalmic **o**utburst syndrome.

To illustrate that sneezing patterns may be inherited—One case study described an individual who always sneezed twice after walking into the sunlight. So did the man's brother and father. And, the 6-month-old daughter carried on the tradition—she sneezed twice when the stroller rolled into the sunlight.

It's hypothesized that there is a selective advantage to being an overly sensitive sneezer. Cold climate populations are constantly exposed to respiratory infections but the frequent sneezers in this group have fewer infections. They forcefully expel the germs before they have a chance to invade the mucosa and take hold.

Just how forceful is the sneeze? The velocity of the sneeze is approximately 100 miles per hour. The velocity of a normal breath is 15 miles per hour. Sneeze particles are propelled 1.5 feet (approximately 100 feet per second). During the first few minutes after a sneeze the bacterial count in the immediate vicinity of the room increases by 500 per cu/mm (cubic millimeter). A single sneeze can carry one million bacteria.

Tripping up the stairs. You can expect to fall or trip up the stairs once every 72,000 times you use them. A researcher from Georgia Tech calls the stairs the most dangerous consumer product after automobiles. This same guy stated that the U.S. has between 1.8 and 2.6 million accidents involving the stairs per year. And just in case you're stressed out about your next stair mishap, remember that more people fall *up* the stairs than down the stairs.

Walking. Most sedentary people take only 3,000 steps per day; however, the total for good health is to accumulate 10,000 steps per day. People with a weight problem should target 15,000 to 18,000 steps per day to lose weight or to maintain weight loss. Two thousand steps is the equivalent of one mile.

Walking *down* the stairs applies a pressure of about seven times your body weight on your kneecap, compared to two times your body weight on walking *up* the stairs.

If you are on a stair-climbing machine in the health club, try not to hold on to the handrails. When holding on to them you shift about 30 pounds of body weight onto the handrails, which in turn decreases energy output by 20 percent.

Walking and blisters. The next time you lace up for a long walk, spray or roll-on antiperspirant on your feet. In a study of West Point cadets, only 21 percent of those who applied it to their feet for five days before a 21-kilometer hike developed blisters, compared to 48 percent who used a placebo spray or roll-on. Why? Less perspiration means less friction, less friction means fewer blisters. Smart thinking.

Walking and erectile dysfunction (ED). Hey, what's a blister or two when the consequences of *not* walking could result in impotence, or erectile dysfunction? Perhaps you're wondering what walking has to do with erections? The Massachusetts Male Aging study has just reported that there is an increased risk of erectile dysfunction in males who burned less than 200 calories per day with exercise. Taking a brisk 20-minute 2-mile walk every day keeps the Viagra away. So, grab those Nikes, roll on the Ban, and start walking.

Yotta Yotta Yotta. Millions used to seem like a huge number to most of us, especially when the number was describing monetary amounts. Heck, millionaires are a dime a dozen these days, as are billionaires. Now that the computer age has hit, even larger numbers are needed to describe computer bytes and computer moguls. The prefix *peta* now applies to quadrillions, *exa* will give you quintillions in your bank account, and *zetta* will be used for sextillions. The highest number described today is *yotta*—used to describe septillions. Bill Gates will most likely be our first yotta-aire.

> *We trained hard, we performed well...but it seemed every time we were beginning to form up into teams and become reasonably proficient we would be reorganized. I was to learn later in life that we tend to meet any one situation by reorganizing...and a wonderful method it can be for creating the illusion of progress while producing confusion, inefficiency and demoralization.*
> —Petronius Arbiter, 210 B.C.

Chapter 3

Gender Benders

> *The only time a woman succeeds in changing a man is when he's a baby.*
> —Natalie Wood (1938-1981)

Myth #1. Men and women are created equal.

Wrong. Mother Nature tends to favor her own when it comes to longevity, with women living 4 to 7 years longer than men. However, Mother Nature doesn't favor her own in the beginning. Male embryos outnumber female embryos by 115 to 100. Unfortunately, the higher rates of stillbirths and miscarriages of males whittle this number to 105 males at birth. Boys also have a higher death rate during infancy and the first six months of life and the male edge continues to decline during adolescence due to a higher number of accidents and homicides. By age 30 all numbers are equal and by age 90 there are nine women for every one male.

Myth #2. Since women live longer they must be healthier.

Well, not exactly. Yes, women do live longer; however, they live with more chronic diseases such as diabetes, arthritis, and Alzheimer's disease than men. Women spend twice as much money on health care as men do, consult physicians more frequently, spend more days in hospitals and have more operations. Obviously obstetrical issues play a role in this gender difference, but when pregnancy and child-care related issues are factored out, women still have the advantage of living longer.

> *Men have a much better time of it than women; for one thing, they marry later; for another thing they die earlier.*
> —H.L.Mencken (1880-1956)

Myth #3. Diamonds are a girl's best friend.

Wrong. Estrogen is. Estrogen performs over 300 functions in the female body. Since most U.S. women are living almost 30 years after their ovaries die, why in the world would we think that this hormone is not important? If your thyroid died at 50, (which it does 8 to 10 times more often in women than it does in men), would you consider going through the rest of your life without thyroid replacement? If, per chance, the testicles bit the dust at 50, could you fathom the primal outbursts if the slightest suggestion were made to not replace the big **T**? Now that should elicit a loud guffaw from the peanut gallery.

Myth #4. The federal government has studied women as vigorously as it has studied men.

Not. The federal government didn't know there were women to study until 1991. Until Bernadine Healy, the first female physician to be the director of the National Institutes of Health, women were virtually ignored as worthy subjects of health-related studies. Actually, the prevailing theory was that women were either barefoot and pregnant or menstruating and miserable and that either of these "female conditions" would throw the study out of kilter. Prior to Dr. Healy, the majority of the government studies were done in their own private laboratories known

Live a Little, Laugh a Lot

as Veteran's Administration Hospitals. The study subjects were essentially 170-pound Caucasian males in their 40s and 50s. Hardly fits the general profile of the population today. Women make up 54 percent of the population, African-Americans comprise 14 percent of the population, and Hispanics are the fastest growing percentage of the population today. Update your data, Uncle Sam.

The egg and the sperm. The female egg is 1,000 times larger than the male sperm. When I took my first human anatomy and physiology class about a millennium ago, the sperm was Dudley Dooright, the male aggressor, and the egg was the poor damsel in distress, bound to the railroad tracks as the locomotive chugged relentlessly forward. Dudley was portrayed as the savior, pounding on his chest, bellowing, "Here I come to save the day!" as the damsel in distress cried, "Help me, help me, Dudley darling!" Well that entire scenario has been canned and the whole truth, and nothing but the truth is as follows: The sperm is *not* the aggressor; the egg is. The egg puckers up and sends out a signal that tells the sperm not only when to swim up the 5-inch Fallopian tube, but also which side to choose. Her signal equals the decibel level of an air raid siren between the ages of 18 and 30, with the peak blast at age 24. By the time she hits her mid-30s the signal becomes weaker and weaker. By the time she reaches 50 she barely even puckers. The implications of this waning whistle are clear—if you can't signal the sperm to swim up the tube, the chances of fertilization diminish. Women in their 40s and 50s have a helluva' time getting pregnant for this reason.

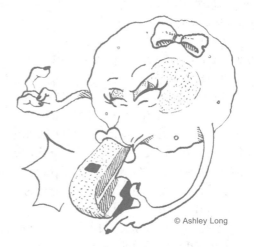

© Ashley Long

The ovary is the most precisely and quantitatively doomed organ in the human body. It is preprogrammed to degenerate at a certain rate, starting before birth. This preprogrammed degeneration has absolutely no regard for race, ethnicity, or religious affiliation. It doesn't take into account your geographic location. The ovary will degenerate precisely at the same time whether you live in Peoria, Illinois, or Perth, Australia. This preprogrammed dropout of eggs has not changed since medical records of women's reproductive status have been kept—over 2,000 years.

At five to six months' gestation, each ovary contains 3.5 million eggs, for a grand total of 7 million eggs. Reflect on this number for just a moment. This horrifying thought means you have the potential for either 7 million children or 7 million periods. Take your pick. Fortunately the ovary has a mind of its own and thinks the exact same thing.

Starting at six months' gestation the ovary undergoes a preprogrammed dropout of eggs known as apoptosis (pronounced a-POH-tosis). During the last trimester of pregnancy the ovaries will lose a grand total of 6.6 million of the original 7 million eggs. At birth the ovaries have a combined 400,000 eggs between them. Whew! This is much more reasonable. You only have to worry about 400,000 children or 400,000 periods. The eggs continue to drop out at a preprogrammed rate so that by the time the young lady reaches 30, there are only 100,000 eggs left—50,000 per ovary. By age 50 the woman has exactly *three* eggs left—count 'em, three.

Don't forget that these eggs are as old as she is, so if she's 52 years old, her eggs are 52 years old. A 52-year-old egg may be considered an old egg, but it's an egg that is still looking for love in *all* the wrong places. Could a 52-year-old woman get pregnant? What are the chances? If she has unprotected sex for two weeks, five times a day (uh-huh like that is really going to happen), her chance of becoming pregnant is less than 1 percent.

So, what about the male half of the deal? Women have all of the eggs they will *ever* possess by the time they are born. Do men have all of the sperm they're going to get at birth? No, men produce sperm *until the day they die*. In fact, they can be brain dead with a flat EEG and heart dead with a flat ECG, and still be pumpin' out one more sperm for the old gipper. Freshly ejaculated sperm is only a little over two months old—75 days old to be exact.

The only difference between the sperm of a 20-year-old male and a 70-year-old male is the rapidity with which the sperm swims. Sperm from the 20-year-old can swim up the 5-inch Fallopian tube in 50 minutes. Sperm from the 70-year-old male gets ejaculated, huffs and puffs, and whines, "You mean I gotta swim now?" It takes 2½ days for the sperm from a 70-year-old to swim up the 5-inch Fallopian tube…gasping, wheezing and snarling on a walker all the way up the tube. The last inch or so is the killer. Once it reaches the egg it gasps "Eureka!" with its last breath and drops dead.

Let's now say you have a 50-year-old female and her partner is a 50-year-old male. His sperm is only 2½ months old, whereas her egg is 50 years old. Let's consider the scenario. How happy is a 50-year-old egg to see a panting, slobbery, oh-so-eager 2½-month-old sperm? Fuggitaboutit.

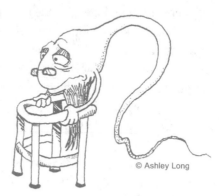

© Ashley Long

Advice for the fertilized egg—"Move it or lose it!" The fertilized egg (the conceptus) has between 6 and 12 days to travel down the 5-inch Fallopian tube and safely implant into the uterine lining. Researchers in the June 10, 1999 *New England Journal of Medicine* followed 189 women after conception. In almost all of the women, the egg implanted 6 to 12 days after ovulation. The later the time of implantation, the more likely the fetus will not survive the first six weeks. In fact, any conceptus implanting after the first 12 days did not produce a live birth in this study.

Why? It appears as if the uterine wall becomes less receptive to implantation later in the menstrual cycle. Another possibility is that fertilized eggs that take a long time to reach the uterus may have defects that make them less likely to survive. Or perhaps both factors contribute to its demise after 12 days of wandering around and looking for love.

Ovulation and conception. When is the best time for the egg and the sperm to meet in the Fallopian tube? The latest research, from the

December 2002 issue of *Obstetrics and Gynecology*, suggests that the very best time to have sex in order to conceive is the day *before* a woman ovulates, *not* the day of ovulation, as previously assumed, and certainly not the day after. In fact, having sex for five straight days, every day before ovulation will give you the best chances of conceiving. This slight change in the recommended day to "do it" might just help 25 percent of the couples that are having problems with conception.

Easier said than done because the first question that comes to mind is: "How the heck do I know when the day *before* ovulation occurs? Should I do it the old fashioned way and take my temperature?" Nope. The temperature rises once the horse is *out* of the barn so to speak, and this might be just one day too late. So put this book down, hop in the car and head to your local drug store. There are over-the-counter kits available for predicting ovulation.

Ovulation and gender behavior. Have you noticed that your suave and debonair husband tends to become quite the Casanova, showering you with love and affection right about the time you ovulate? Guys are more likely to call you more, wonder what you're doing, where you are, how you're feeling—behavior known as *monopolization* when you are most fertile. In fact, research from a University of New Mexico study reported an increase of 30 percent in this type of behavior around the time of ovulation.

In contrast, women become less interested in their mate, and are more likely to fantasize about other partners as well as cheating on their partner just before ovulation. In other words, that UPS guy is looking awfully handsome as the egg prepares for ejection from the ovary. "What husband? Of course, I'm single."

Researchers are calling this discrepancy in behaviors between the two sexes as a "conflict of interest." Well *hello*. Woman instinctively want to have sex with as many partners as possible in order to ensure the genetic quality of their offspring, whereas men are more interested in "me, me, me." They want to make sure that only their genes get the big prize. (Steven Gangestad, University of New Mexico)

Smell and ovulation. Peak smelling ability occurs between the ages of 30 and 50 and declines steadily afterwards. Women have a much keener sense of smell than men as well as better tasting abilities. Estrogen gives females their edge when it comes to enjoying a greater sense of smell. A female can detect musk, the scent associated with male bodies, better than any other odor. When estrogen levels peak during ovulation, a woman's smell is most acute and can detect musk 100 to 100,000 times more keenly than during menstruation. Teleologically this would appear to be a reproductive advantage for obvious reasons. Researchers from the Monell Chemical Senses Center in Philadelphia think that estrogen may affect either the olfactory cells in the nose, which also have estrogen receptors, or it may exert its effect via higher cognitive functions, like learning and memory.

> *Have you ever dated someone because you were too lazy to commit suicide?*
> —Judy Tenuta

This gender difference may also explain why women are more intolerant of environmental odors and file more complaints concerning foul odors. It may also explain why women suffer from more chemical insensitivities and "sick building syndrome."

What is your preference when looking for a date, a mate, or a relationship?
Percentage of women who look at a man's face first: 56
Percentage of men who look at a woman's face first: 60

Percentage of women who look at a man's eyes first: 21
Percentage of men who look at a woman's eyes first: 4
(The obvious question is what *do* men look at first?)

Percentage of women who prefer blue eyes in men: 52
Percentage of men who prefer blue eyes in women: 38

Percentage of women who prefer blond men: 17
Percentage of men who prefer blond women: 35

MOUSE PERSONALS

SBF (single, brown, female) ISO (in search of) SBM (single, brown, male) for an intense, impersonal, one-night stand. Objective—superior babies that are capable of resisting parasites and other diseases. Long walks on the beach aren't necessary…your place or mine? Please reply with scratch 'n sniff urine-scented card. Photo not necessary.

The female rodent is quite picky about choosing her mate, and she chooses her mate in a most peculiar way. She uses the old schnoz to smell the urine scent of a prospective partner. Why? A portion of the MHC (major histocompatibility complex) is excreted in the urine. (The MHC complex is a group of genes that not only establishes tissues as "self versus non-self," but also codes for the animal's immune response to foreign "non-self" tissue.) The female is seeking a male with certain genes that will best complement her own. The end result is that she avoids inbreeding and she will produce offspring that are more genetically diverse and more disease-resistant. This of course, continues to propagate the species and a healthier one at that. Why can't humans be as intuitive as rodents? (*Discover,* June 1992)

Living together and looking alike. Why do people who live together long enough start to look alike? Is it their diet? Is it the weather? Is it in the water? Is it because they married their cousin Susie? None of the above, it appears. Researchers at the University of Michigan attribute the shared resemblance to having similar emotional experiences over the years. Therefore, they tend to reflect each other's facial expressions in what is referred to as "repeated empathic mimicry." The theory is that similar facial expressions will sculpt similar faces. An additional implication of this theory is that your kids may look like you not only because of genetics, but also as the result of repeated empathic mimicry.

Muscle mass and gender differences. Muscle mass is lost at a rate of 4 to 6 percent per decade starting at age 40 in women and age 60 in men. However, after only two months of strength training, women recover a decade of loss and men recover two decades. (William Evans, University of Arkansas for Medical Sciences)

Men and mutations. In a recent study published in the journal *Nature,* genetic mutations occur 5.25 times more often in males than females. Researchers found that the mutations were not caused by environmental effects but by random errors that occur when a person's DNA divides.

Crying and gender. Why is it that women are prone to cry more often than men? The quivering bottom lip, the moist eyes, the rapid blinking and the sniffling nose are seen much more often in the female sex. It's probably due to the presence of a certain hormone and *not* social conditioning. The hormone responsible for this annoying phenomenon is prolactin (pro—to promote, lactin—lactation). Prolactin is found in the serum of both sexes; however, women have 60 percent more prolactin than men. Prior to puberty, boys and girls have equal amounts of prolactin in their serum and cry equally as often. When puberty rears its ugly head, prolactin levels decline in males (why would a man need to lactate?) and prolactin levels increase in females, to prepare for lactation at some point in the near or distant future.

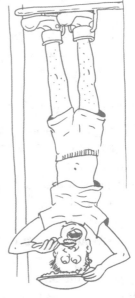

Speaking of crying—did you know? Tears drain down into the throat even when the body is hanging upside down.

Hormonal changes during pregnancy in the fathers-to-be. Well, how does this happen? Who's pregnant here? Of course hormones would be changing in the pregnant female preparing her for the numerous changes that occur during the nine months as well as the changes that are necessary for delivery. But why in the world would hormonal changes occur in the expectant father? Canadian researchers found that hormonal

© Frank Salcido

changes occurring in the serum in pregnant mothers can be mimicked in saliva. To examine hormonal changes occurring in the fathers-to-be, Canadian researchers collected saliva in 45 men who accompanied their wives to the prenatal exams. They started collecting saliva early in pregnancy and continued collecting saliva every week. The big surprise— hormonal levels in the expectant fathers became more like that of their wives during the last three weeks of the pregnancy. In other words, the father's testosterone levels plummeted, while their estrogen and prolactin levels increased. Their cortisol levels also rose during the week prior to birth, probably in order to help them cope more easily with the stress of their wife's pregnancy—*yeah, right.* The researchers speculated that these changes most likely helped prepare the dads mentally for fatherhood and, it is thought, may help them assist with child rearing and domestic affairs. Uh-huh. (*Mayo Clinic Proceedings* 2001; 76:582)

Pregnancy makes fathers fat and drunk. First-time fathers gain an average of 3.5 pounds during their spouse's pregnancy. Not only do they pack the food away, they also swill down the booze. Researchers at the Flinders Medical Center in Adelaide, Australia blame the booze and the flab on the stress and depression that accompany the life style changes associated with pregnancy. Husbands feel neglected in many areas, but the greatest stress is associated with the lack of intimacy. About 40 percent of the first time dads said they had sex less frequently than they expected during the pregnancy and after the baby was born. Their only consolation was food and the bottle—and not the baby bottle.

Nicotine and gender. The effect of nicotine on mood varies greatly between the sexes. In women, nicotine has a calming effect, an antidepressant effect, and it reduces aggression. In men, it provokes aggression and triggers anxiety. This difference may be one reason women find it more difficult than men to stop smoking. (Fili S. British Pharmacologic Society Meeting, London, March 2001)

Alcohol consumption and gender differences. Males have traditionally held the number one spot in the race for the most alcoholics. However, the 3:1 male-to-female ratio for alcoholism is narrowing as more women, especially young women, are experiencing more serious problems with alcohol. A survey conducted by the Gallup Organization reports there are 4.5 million women with a drinking problem, 2.5 million who consume at least 60 drinks per month. The alcoholic beverage most frequently consumed by women is wine and the average age at which women start drinking is 13.

Besides the obvious physical differences between males and females, alcoholism is a greater problem physiologically for women than it is for men. Women become intoxicated more easily due to 30 percent less gastric alcohol dehydrogenase, an enzyme located in the stomach lining that metabolizes alcohol. Since there is less of this enzyme in women, alcohol is absorbed directly through the stomach lining without being metabolized into a more *inactive* metabolite. The active form of alcohol is more directly toxic to the female heart and liver. As a result, women are twice as likely to die of alcoholism-related illnesses such as cirrhosis of the liver and an enlarged heart known as cardiomyopathy as male drinkers of the same age. In addition, the incidence of cirrhosis and cardiomyopathy occurs a full 10 years prior to that of men.

This is a double-edged sword for women. The good news is that moderate drinking, defined as one drink per day for a woman, appears to protect against stroke, Alzheimer's disease, and reduce the risk of heart disease. The bad news is that one drink per day slightly increases the risk of breast cancer due to the metabolism of alcohol into estrogen-like substances by the liver.

The good news again is that a new study of 90,000 women demonstrates that for women who drink one to two drinks a day and also take more than 300 mcg (0.3 mg) of folic acid per day, the risk of breast cancer reverts to that of a nondrinker. Folic acid is essential for DNA synthesis, and unfortunately alcohol blocks the absorption of folic acid. Taking more than 300 mcg (0.3 mg) overrides the absorption problem, enabling women to maintain its cancer-protective properties. So if you drink, check your multivitamin and make sure it contains at least 300 mcg (0.3 mg) of folic acid.

Depression and gender differences. Because differences in the prevalence of depression between men and women apply only to adults and do not emerge until adolescence, a number of researchers have studied the period of adolescence to determine why females are more likely to

> *When women are depressed they either eat or go shopping. Men invade another country.*
> –Elayne Boosler

be depressed than males. Research has focused on the hormonal changes that occur during puberty as predisposing factors for gender-related depression.

With the onset of menses at puberty, the female brain is exposed to monthly surges of estrogen and progesterone. Both estrogen and progesterone may influence mood and behavior by affecting neurotransmitter synthesis, release, reuptake, and enzymatic deactivation. Estrogen has been shown to control the levels of two neurotransmitters responsible for happiness and energy production. The neurotransmitters are serotonin and norepinephrine. Estrogen not only boosts the production of both neurotransmitters but it also decreases the enzyme that degrades each neurotransmitter. Progesterone has been shown to increase the breakdown of the two neurotransmitters, resulting in decreased levels of both neurotransmitters and a lack of energy and depression.

The incidence of depression is greater during a woman's reproductive years; however, in adults over age 55 there is a clear reversal in the prevalence of depression, resulting in a higher incidence of depression in men. This supports the hypothesis that the increased incidence of depression in females may be a phenomenon of reproductive years.

Before the age of 11, the incidence of depression either does not differ between genders, or is slightly higher in boys, again supporting the hypothesis that puberty plays a major role in the emergence of depression. The appearance of gender differences in depression first occurs between the ages of 13 and 15 years and the greatest increase occurs between the ages of 15 and 18 years.

Psychosocial theories for the emergence of depression during adolescence include acute stressors, such as sexual abuse during childhood and battery and rape during adulthood. The overall rates for sexual abuse increase significantly for girls between the ages of 10 and 14 years, and girls and adolescents are two to three times more likely to be the victims of sexual abuse than males. Research suggests that the increase in sexual abuse occurring in early adolescence leads directly to more depression in females and to the gender differences in depression that emerge at that time.

PET (postitron emission tomography) scans and depression. PET scanners track a radioisotope that concentrates in physiologically activated areas of the brain. When researchers asked patients to think really sad thoughts, an area in the frontal cortex, known as the orbital frontal cortex, was activated. An interesting gender difference was observed. In sad women the orbital frontal cortex was activated on both sides of the brain, whereas activity in depressed men was only observed on the left frontal cortex. Could this explain why depression is more common in women? Or is it just the fact that women have a bigger corpus collosum connecting the two hemispheres and women tend to share brain activity between the two hemispheres more than men do.

Another interesting gender difference is the ability to distinguish emotions on someone else's face. Both men and women were equally adept at distinguishing a happy face. And women had no trouble distinguishing sadness in men and women's faces. Men, however, could distinguish if a man's face was depressed but had absolutely no clue when trying to determine if a woman was depressed. A woman's face had to be *really* sad for a male to recognize their sadness. So much for recognizing subtle nuances of emotion.

Brain differences and sexual identity. Now here's a can of worms that has been opened slightly but needs to be opened a bit more. The new functional MRIs (magnetic resonance imaging) are able to determine structure and function of various parts of the body with electrifying accuracy. When evaluating a small area at the base of the brain known as the hypothalamus, a consistent structural difference between the genders is the size of the preoptic nucleus. This area is quite large in the male and significantly smaller in the female. What is the function of this nucleus?

The preoptic nucleus produces two hormones, ADH (antidiuretic hormone) and oxytocin. The primary function of ADH is to regulate free water balance and maintain serum osmolality; however, it has been shown to play a role in memory acquisition (especially during sleep) and in sexual behavior and mating. Oxytocin stimulates uterine contraction during orgasm and assists with the milk letdown response necessary for breast-feeding.

Based on the function of these two hormones, many neuroscientists postulate that the preoptic nucleus may play a role in sexual function, sexual behavior, and sexual orientation. This difference is postulated to be the result of intrauterine testosterone production by the male fetus.

This hypothesis has surely stimulated heated discussions amongst the experts in the fields of neurology, psychology, sociology, theology and any other "ology" that might want to throw their two cents in. In other words, the heated discussions cover topics including the origins of sexuality, sexual orientation and behavior, and gender identity. Does each individual have a specific sexual orientation that is 100 percent predetermined by the size of the preoptic nucleus? If you have a large preoptic nucleus do you identify with male sexual behavior, whether you are a male or female? Do gay men have a smaller preoptic nucleus than straight men? Do gay women have a larger preoptic nucleus than straight women, especially if they have masculine tendencies? Is the size of the preoptic nucleus determined by the amount of testosterone the fetal brain was exposed to prenatally or is this determined by environmental influences? If you can answer all of these questions you will be the next Nobel Prize winner in all of the fields ending in "ology."

Dr. Simon LeVay of the Scripps Institute has been trying to answer these questions and more. He has compared the size of the preoptic nucleus in gay men, who had succumbed to the complications of HIV and AIDS, with straight men who had died from other causes. He found that gay men had smaller preoptic nucleuses than heterosexual men; however, he could not determine if this was truly a biologic difference present from fetal development or if the changes occurred after birth as a result of environmental influences *or* if the changes were due to the disease process. He did establish that the preoptic nucleus was the same size in all of the gay men. It was comparable to the size of the preoptic nucleus in heterosexual women. Is anyone confused yet? What does all of this mean? Nothing at the moment, but stay tuned. You may be checking out the size of your preoptic nucleus in the future prior to checking out the opposite or same sex.

Behavior and gender differences. Brain imaging studies from the University of Pennsylvania School of Medicine observed the metabolic activity of the brains of 37 young men and 24 young women at rest. They were asked to just let their minds free associate and not think of any particular subject.

A major difference was noted between the genders. Men had higher metabolic activity in the area of the brain known as the limbic system. The limbic system is the most primitive area of the deep cerebral cortex and it is responsible for our most primitive behaviors and emotions. This area is also the "autonomic" or "automatic" nervous system and it is involved with the immediate response to situations. In other words, you don't have to think and analyze your response, the limbic system just responds. So as a consequence, you act before you think. Women, in contrast, demonstrated higher metabolic activity in the more evolved and complex areas combining the anterior limbic system with the higher cortical functioning or the analytic portion of the brain.

In other words, to simplify the issue, the male brain activity was centered in the "action" area of the limbic system and the female brain activity was concentrated in the "symbolic" area of higher cortical function. A simple analogy might help explain this difference.

If a dog is angry and jumps up and bites you, that is an action. However, if the dog is angry and he bares his teeth and growls, that is more symbolic behavior. In human behavior a man might ram his fist through the wall or kick the side of a tire if he is angry. The woman would growl and bare her teeth. Just kidding. The woman might say "Oh, I'm feeling upset about this behavior." And, her facial expressions and body language would provide the symbolic message.

Sex and the septagenarian. It appears as if Americans don't slow down when it comes to doing the "big nasty." An Arizona retirement community recently had to send a bulletin out to all of its residents (both male and female residents) reminding them that golf courses, parks and swimming pools were *not* appropriate settings for "coupling," as it were.

Sex in the tube, and not in the test tube. Modern technology has become a scientific bedroom of sorts. A gynecologist from the Netherlands persuaded eight couples to make love inside the tube of an MRI (magnetic resonance image) scanner. The scanner recorded the physiologic changes in all of the couples from the first touch to the last push. Dr. Weijmar Schultz discovered some intriguing findings concerning both genders. First of all, while in the missionary position, the male penis is shaped much like a boomerang. (Brings to mind a song, "My boomerang won't come back, my boomerang won't come back.") One might wonder why this physiologic adaptation occurred, and Dr. Schultz is still wondering the same thing as well. And, wondering why his boomerang won't come back.

The second finding was that the uterus does not double in size during sexual activity, refuting the findings of the sex gurus of the past, Masters and Johnson. In their defense, however, Masters and Johnson did not have an MRI scanner at their disposal when they were observing

Historical Highlights

In the year 1884, a surgeon from a Baltimore ENT hospital, Dr. John Noland Mackenzie, reconfirmed an earlier medical theory that the nose and genitals had a close relationship. He was the first to propose that the size of the nose correlated with the size of the penis. He observed that the tissue of the nose had similar erectile tissue as that of the penis and that under conditions of arousal "erection of this tissue" takes place.

Dr. Mackenzie waxed prolific on this issue. He also believed that irritation of the nose could reflexly cause irritation of the genital organs. The corollary here being that chronic masturbation might produce chronic nasal problems. Could this explain the increased incidence of chronic sinusitis in this country?

He also commented on a supposed swelling of the nasal mucosa during menses and postulated the existence of a "vicarious nasal menstruation," meaning that a nosebleed might replace or supplant menstruation. (It is a known fact that nosebleeds are statistically more common during menses, however, the vicarious nature of the nosebleed is currently questioned.)

the sex act between couples. They only had their two pairs of eyes, and when observing from an observation booth it is literally impossible to see the shape of the penis or the size of the uterus.

Sleep alone if you want a good night's sleep. "Spooning" your beloved may not be the perfect way to enter la-la land. That's the finding from two research studies from the Loughborough University of Technology in England. Sleep researcher Francesca Pankhurst fitted 46 couples with wristwatch devices that recorded body movements and monitored their sleep for eight nights. She found that almost half of all tossing by one bedmate triggered tossing by the other. In the second study, people slept longer and more peacefully when their partners were away for the night. However, when asked, the majority of the study participants said they slept better *with* their partners than without. Why? Women reported feeling more secure with their partners close by and men, being the ever-so-sensitive gender, said they just weren't used to sleeping alone.

Is marriage a high risk factor for chronic heartburn? Not only is a lousy night of sleep a downside to being married, you can add the high risk of heartburn as well. Of the population of patients with heartburn, 57 percent are married, 13 percent have never been married, 13 percent are divorced, 10 percent are widowed, 3 percent are separated, and 2 percent are living together but not married. Moral of the story? (*American Family Physician,* Sept.15, 1991)

Addendum: According to *American Demographics,* Birmingham, Alabama wins the prize as having the most adults with heartburn—72 percent of the population of this city is popping H2 blockers (Tagamet, Pepcid, Zantac,or Axid) or

> *Blood transfusion is like marriage; it should not be entered in upon lightly, unadvisably or wantonly, or more often than is absolutely necessary.*
> —Anonymous

proton pump inhibitors (Prilosec, Nexium, Prevacid, Protonix, or Aciphex).

Loving your car. A 1994 Wall Street Journal survey on the importance of the automobile disclosed a few interesting facts. Thirty-eight percent of the men surveyed loved their car more than they loved their women. Eight percent of the women surveyed said they found men who drive spiffy cars much more appealing than men who pulled up in a Yugo. Fifteen percent of the population named their cars. The most popular names were "Betsy," "My Baby," and "Angel."

Stop and smell the roses—especially if you're in pain. The sweet smell of roses may alter the brain's chemistry, making a woman more able to tolerate pain. A study from researchers at the University of Québec asked 20 women and 20 men to hold one of their hands in painfully hot water for as long as possible while sniffing different scents. When women smelled pleasant odors such as roses or almonds they stated that their pain was tolerable for longer periods of time. When they smelled foul odors such as vinegar, their pain worsened. This same scenario did not hold true for the men in the study. The smells did not have any effect on the perceived intensity of pain in this group. It appears as if smells alter the sensory processing of touch and pain in female brains but not male brains.

Overeating on the first date. Women who pig out on a dinner date will probably *not* be asked out for dinner again by that same dinner partner. Researchers have found that women who eat like birds, are perceived (by both men and women) as more feminine and better looking than those who eat heartily. On the other hand, a measure of masculinity is how well the guy can pack it away at a meal. So he can wolf it down, while she demurely picks at her Caesar salad, with the dressing on the side, of course.

Bathroom facilities. A study of highway rest stops in the state of Washington revealed that males averaged 45 seconds in the rest room compared to females who averaged 79 seconds. The female researcher reporting this vital gender difference came to the startling conclusion that the 50:50 ratio between women and men's toilet facilities in public rest rooms around the country was unfair. How many times have you reached the same conclusion when standing in line at a movie theater, ballgame, or concert?

Vocal cords. How do we produce sounds? Our vocal cords, which are thick, tough folds of connective tissue and ligament, produce sounds by vibrating as exhaled air puffs through them. The vibrations are extremely rapid—125 cycles per second in men, 200 cycles per second in women. Differences in length and thickness of vocal folds largely account for the contrast in frequency, which our ears perceive as pitch. In men, the folds are typically 7/8th to 1¼ inches long. In women, they're ¼-inch shorter on average and half as thick. Consequently, men have a lower voice. Testosterone, by the way, is responsible for enlarging and thickening of the vocal cords.

Coital noise pollution. Noisy lovemaking can be even more stressful to the folks in the room next door or the apartment below than a boom box blaring at 110 decibels. However, unlike those neighbors who are quick to complain about the blasting boom box, the neighbors listening to loud lovemaking will generally *not* complain or pound on the door and tell the couple to turn it down a notch.

Orgasmic cephalgia. Well, it looks like disturbing the neighbors isn't the only thing that might result from exuberant and noisy lovemaking. One in 100 men "suffer" from severe headaches that occur just at the moment of orgasm. This is three times more common in the male gender than the female gender and it usually affects men in their 20s. The headache can last weeks, even though the orgasm only lasts seconds. Bummer.

Speed and gender differences. Researchers at the University of Cape Town in South Africa believe that women's marathon times can beat men's in the very near future—this year perhaps. The difference in running speed between the sexes narrows as distance increases. Women are already faster than men in 56-mile ultramarathons.

Intestinal gas and gender. The average person releases between 500 and 2,000 ml of gas per day via the rectum, with an average volume of 90 ml per expulsion for women and an average of 125 ml for men. Note the gender difference with this statistic—one that men are particular proud of on any given expulsion. Yeah, baby.

Before you decide to choose the sex of your child—read this. Giving birth to a boy shortens the mom's life by a whopping 34 weeks, whereas giving birth to a girl actually lengthens a woman's life by 23 weeks, says a study of 375 women who lived in Finland between the seventeenth and nineteenth centuries. The reason: Boys are much more demanding to produce. Why? For one reason, they are usually heavier at birth than girls. For another reason, women pregnant with boys have higher circulating testosterone levels that in turn may suppress the mothers' immune systems. Also, girls may extend the life span of a mom because they typically are more available to help out around the house. (How hard are you laughing at this one, Mom?)

P.S. You might be wondering why this study looked at the life spans of women between the seventeenth and nineteenth centuries. The findings are based on extremely accurate church records and show the effects of natural mortality before the arrival of modern medicine. (S. Helle, University of Turku, Finland)

In a similar study from the National Maternity Hospital in Dublin, researchers found that boys were 20 percent more likely to require instrument-assisted deliveries, and 50 percent more likely to require cesarean sections. They were more likely to be in fetal distress and need serum samples for oxygen deficiency. Boys have larger heads, which may account for the need for instrumentation and C-sections, but the researchers weren't sure of the causes of an increase in fetal distress.

Can what you eat influence the sex of your child? Controversial to say the least, but two researchers in the 1970s postulated that certain combinations of electrolytes could influence the sex of the child. A diet high in sodium and potassium, but low in magnesium and calcium would increase the chances of having a boy, whereas a diet low in sodium and potassium and high in magnesium and calcium would increase the chances of having a girl. Out of 281 pregnancies tested, 83 percent gave birth to babies of the "right" sex. Unfortunately, controlled studies have not yet confirmed the findings.

Blue vs. pink. In ancient times it was believed that evil spirits hovered over nurseries and that these evil spirits could be dispelled by certain colors that were presumed to combat evil. Blue was considered the most powerful color because of its association with the sky and heavenly spirits. Boys in ancient times were considered the most valuable child and blue clothing was considered as valuable. A few hundred years later girls came into a color of their own, pink. It was claimed that baby girls were born inside pink roses and thus the association was made.

Divorce and the gender of the child. A woman who only has a daughter is 9 percent more likely to be separated or divorced than a woman with only a son. In two-child families, marriages were most stable when both children were boys. The risk of a divorce rose 9 percent when one of the two children was a girl and 18 percent when both children were girls. Why, one might ask? University of Pennsylvania researchers found that fathers spend more leisure time with their sons and are more involved in making the rules for their sons. The researchers hypothesize that because of the way men and women are socialized, there are more things for a father to do with a son. Therefore, fathers are drawn more closely into the family unit by having a son.

Allergic reactions during sexual intercourse. Two types of allergic responses can occur during or after sexual intercourse. The two reactions are due to an allergy to seminal fluid and can be either a localized allergic reaction or a systemic reaction known as anaphylaxis. The localized reaction occurs in the female genital tissues and includes burning pain, redness, and swelling. This reaction lasts from 24 to 48 hours after intercourse and is most likely mediated by IgE-type anti-sperm antibodies. This certainly won't kill the woman, but it would certainly be an unwanted side effect after a night between the sheets.

The second type of reaction, anaphylactic shock, is a whole different ballgame. This is a life-threatening emergency situation and causes generalized itching, shortness of breath, low blood pressure and shock.

In other words, two minutes of orgasmic pleasure can put you six feet under.

"Whoa, whoa, whoa!" you shriek. Does this mean that every time you "make-a-love to yo'husband" you have the potential to *die*? Would you feel an impending sense of doom every time he approaches with that little gleam in his eye? Would you have to load up on epinephrine and oxygen to prevent shock—*prior* to doing the big nasty? Are you having rapid respirations from the pleasure you have received from the lovemaking or are you gasping for breath due to widespread bronchoconstriction and impending respiratory failure?

What to do? You "lov'a yo' husband," you wanna "make-a-love to yo' husband," but you don't "wanna die in the arms of yo' husband." Sooooooo—two preventative measures may be undertaken for the above two problems. First of all the use of condoms can prevent both the localized allergic reaction and the generalized anaphylactic reaction. The condom prevents contact between the vaginal membranes and the seminal fluid. However, if condoms aren't an option, the original idea of epinephrine and oxygen by the bedside is your only other alternative. Remember this—a shot of epinephrine lasts for 15 minutes and *he doesn't!*

Well, then, how long *does* he last? The average length of sexual intercourse for humans is two, yes, I said two, minutes. This doesn't seem like an interminable amount of time but you can thank your lucky stars that you are not a chimpanzee. The average length of intercourse for a chimpanzee is *seven seconds*…uh, huh. Let me repeat that, *seven seconds*.

Sex and the single 3-spined stickleback. Standard evolutionary theory states that the females are generally the choosier of the sexes when it comes to picking a mate. This rationale is based on the fact that a female's maximum reproductive output is more limited than

The gender of a crocodile is determined purely by the weather. If it's hot outside it's a boy; if it's cold, it's a girl.

a male's. Eggs are more costly to make than sperm and the female's number of descendants is limited to the number of eggs she can produce while a male's posterity depends more on the absolute number of females he can mate with.

Let's take a look at your everyday, average 3-spined stickleback for example:

The male develops a bright red belly when he is ready to mate. This signals the female that he is ready and "lookin' for love." When the female sees his "badge" of maleness, she moseys on over to inspect him and the nest that he has built for "the kids." If she approves, she deposits her eggs in the nest and he fertilizes them immediately.

Her approval of him as a mate is based on just *how red* his belly is. The judgment is based on the fact that the depth of color is a good indicator of how free a male is of parasitic infection and therefore of how good a father he will be. If a male stickleback cannot produce the accepted amount of the pigment, then he obviously won't have what it takes to make a good father. The red belly is not a badge of courage, it is an honest signal of health.

As you can imagine, the male stickleback with the reddest belly is the most popular guy in town. In fact, numerous female sticklebacks court him so he has the liberty of being rather picky in choosing his mate. He rules the nest, nurtures the eggs, and would therefore prefer healthy eggs. As a rule of thumb in the stickleback world of choosing eggs, the heavier the egg, the healthier it is, and the more likely it will breed a healthy baby stickleback. The size of the female stickleback correlates with the weight of her eggs; therefore, he chooses the heaviest of the females.

House husbands and heart attacks. If you have decided to become a house husband and let your wife "bring home the bacon," you might want to think again. A recent study by Eaker Epidemiology Enterprises in Wisconsin studied 2,682 people between 18 and 77 for 10 years and found that men who do all of the housework, chores, child care and cleaning have an *82 percent* higher death rate than guys who get up every morning and head to the office. Now, that's a jaw dropper. The implication is clear. Stay-at-home dads may become much more stressed about the role reversal and how others perceive them. In addition, since

> *The best cure for hypochondria is to forget about your body and get interested in someone else's.*
> — Goodman Ace
> 1899-1982

house husbands are few and far between, the lack of social support from the guys increases the stress level. One other major reason might be the fact that men just aren't prepared for the task of caring for a family. Many assume that it's a piece of cake—like what's the big deal? How hard can it be? Once they realize all of the skills and "multi-tasking" (the big buzzword these days) it involves, their stress levels skyrocket. "How can I get all of this done, and the kids picked up before Hillary gets home?"

We even laugh differently. When it comes to laughter, the girls giggle and the guys grunt. Jo-Anne Bachorowski, an acoustical scientist from Vanderbilt University, studied 97 volunteers. She asked them to watch various film clips and secretly taped their laughter. The segments included the fake orgasm scene in the movie *When Harry Met Sally* and the "bring out the dead scene" from the film *Monty Python's Holy Grail*. After evaluating the various sounds, Dr. Bachorowski concluded that women were more likely to produce "voiced," or songlike laughs such as giggles and chuckles, while men were more likely to grunt and snort. Once again, no surprise here.

Fat cells and gender differences. The fat cells of a 120-pound female can store an extra 74,000 calories; those from a 160-pound man can store an extra 95,000 calories. (Remember, 3,500 calories = 1 pound.) Women increase their body fat by 26 percent per decade of age, whereas men only increase

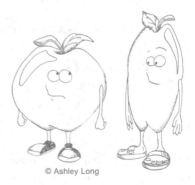

© Ashley Long

their body fat content by 17 percent with each decade of age. Now, where is the Equal Rights Amendment (ERA) when we need it?

Not your ordinary sex-change operation. A husband and wife in Beijing exchanged sex organs in a 19-hour operation. Wouldn't you think that if your partner wants to change sex organs that the marriage might be over? Well, obviously not if you are both changing in the opposite direction. Husband Wang received wife Hou's female parts, and wife Hou received Wang's male organs in a true scenario of Hou Wanged Who? They then exchanged names, exchanged outfits, remained married and lived happily ever after.

Dr. Tatiana's take on gender differences. After all is said and done, and this chapter has been completed, we all know that stereotypical men and women may actually be the exception rather than the rule. We can see ourselves in both roles—some of us gals hog the remote, some guys don't prefer blondes. Well, maybe that's not a great example. But let's just say that gender stereotypes are fun to learn and to observe, but also remember Dr. Tatiana's words of wisdom:

> When you gaze at a couple and wonder
> What trait makes him "him" and her "her,"
> Beware, for it's easy to blunder
> And be false in what you aver.

> Some creatures change sex before teatime,
> Some others find two sexes dull,
> And that virile male fish has no free time—
> He's got all his kiddies to lull.

> When it comes to the topic of gender,
> Mother Nature's been having some fun.
> Take nothing for granted! Remember,
> You won't find any rules—not a one!

(Judson, O. *Dr. Tatiana's Sex Advice to All Creation*. Metropolitan Books, Henry Holt and Company, New York, NY, 2002)

He said, she said

He said, *I don't know why you bother wearing a bra—you have nothing to put in it.*

She said, *You wear pants, don't you?*

Chapter 4

Sugar and Spice & Everything Nice

> *Can you imagine a world without men? No crime and lots of happy fat women.*
> —Nicole Hollander

Who put the "men" in menstruate? Many feminist writers have taken umbrage against the sexist English language. They have vowed to change the "no-MEN-cla-ture" not only in everyday language, such as in *mail person* and *womyn*, but also in the medical field. Keeping all of these important changes in mind I came across this little ditty:

I wonder if our new estate
will alter nature's laws
Will wopersons personstruate
until personopause
Anonymous

Well then, where did the "men" come from? Menstruate, menses, menarche (the onset of puberty and periods), menorrhagia (heavy menstrual flow); amenorrhea means without periods; Amen (the prefix "A" in medicine means "without" so Amen must mean without men);—Amen. *Men*- is the prefix taken from the Greek *mēn,* meaning a month, and *mēnē,* "the moon." The cyclic changes in the moon provided one of the earliest measures of time, about 29½ days—just about the same amount of time between the cyclical bleeding in women. In Latin, a month is *mensis* with the plural *menses,* and *menstruus* means "monthly." Colloquially, some women still refer to their "monthlies" and since they occur predictably in most women, they have also been referred to as periods. The menopause obviously means the party is over—or a cessation of menses (*pausis* is the Greek term for "cessation.") (Haubrich WS, *Medical Meanings*, Harcourt Brace Jovanovich, Publishers, New York, 1984.)

If *men* could *me*nstruate. The following excerpts are from Gloria Steinem's essay titled "If men could menstruate." The entire text of the essay can be found in Gloria Steinem's book, *Outrageous Acts and Everyday Rebellions* (1983).

…So what would happen if suddenly, magically, men could menstruate and women could not?

Clearly, menstruation would become an enviable, boast worthy, masculine event:

Men would brag about how much and how long.

Young boys would talk about it as the envied beginning of manhood. Gifts, religious ceremonies, family dinners, and stag parties would mark the day.

To prevent monthly work loss among the powerful, Congress would fund a National Institute of Dysmenorrhea. Doctors would research little about heart attacks, from which men were hormonally protected, but everything about cramps.

Sanitary supplies would be federally funded and free. Of course, some men would still pay for the prestige of such commercial brands as Paul Newman Tampons, Muhammad Ali's Rope-a-Dope Pads, John Wayne Maxi Pads, and Joe Namath Jock Shields—"For Those Light Bachelor Days."

Statistical surveys would show that men did better in sports and won more Olympic medals during their periods.

Generals, right-wing politicians, and religious fundamentalists would cite menstruation ("*men*-struation") as proof that only men could serve God and country in combat ("You have to give blood to take blood"), occupy high political office ("Can women be properly fierce without a monthly cycle governed by the planet Mars?"), be priests, ministers, God Himself ("He gave his blood for our sins"), or rabbis ("Without a monthly purge of impurities, women are unclean").

...TV shows would treat the subject openly. (*Happy Days:* Richie and Potsie try to convince Fonzie that he is still "The Fonz" even though he has missed two periods in a row. *Hill Street Blues:* The whole precinct hits the same cycle).

On your next vacation to Maryland you might want to stop by **The Museum of Menstruation.** It is located in New Carrollton, Maryland, approximately seven miles northeast of Washington D.C. You can give them a quick call ahead of time if you want to drop by. The phone number is 301-459-4450. You can also check out their website at www.mum.org.

Menstruating elephant shrews. The only non-primates known to naturally menstruate are the elephant shrew and one species of bat, the *Glossaphage sorcinia*.

Menstrual synchrony. It's a woman thing. You're working with a group of women and you all start work together on the same day. Nary a one of you has any idea whether or not the other gals in the group are menstruating, nor would it be something you would ask everyone on your first day in the office. However, within three months, as women trickle into work one morning, Susie might say: "Oh mercy, I started my period this morning." Then Helen walks in and moans, "Anyone have a Motrin? I just started my period on the way to work." Betty comes out of the office restroom asking, "Does anyone have an extra tampon? I just started my period." And Candy skips down the hall gleefully exclaiming, "Hallelujah, my period arrived. Whew!" This phenomenon is referred to as menstrual synchrony and it just so happens that as we all work together and are exposed to one another's pheromones, we begin

In an 1879 textbook, an American gynecologist advised girls to "spend the year before and the two years after puberty at rest." In addition, each menstrual period should be endured in the "recumbent position" until the girls' systems could adjust to the "new order of life." Another medical specialist wrote that excessive exercise by women would have a negative effect on the "genital organs, for they tend to decay."

to cycle together. (Guys—beware. If we all cycle together it means that we are all premenstrual together too. When PMS hits an entire group of women at the same time things can get *really* ugly.)

Is this really true? Rumor has it that the Israeli Army uses this cycling to its advantage. All of the Israeli Army female soldiers live together in the barracks and all start cycling their periods together. The Israeli Army will only send them out for combat when they are in their premenstrual phase—when they're *really* cranky. If this is a true story it's a brilliant tactical move. Two thousand women with PMS could decimate an opposing military force ten times their size.

Menstrual synchrony and armpit odor. Martha McClintock, a pioneer in studying menstrual "cycling," first reported in the early 1970s that women who lived together or who worked together influenced one another's menstrual cycles. At the time, Dr. McClintock could not explain why that happened, but 25 years later, she and her colleagues have identified the trigger. The trigger just so happens to be located in the armpits.

In Dr. McClintock's study women were exposed to odorless compounds taken from another woman's underarm at various points in her menstrual cycle. They found that exposure to compounds taken from the early stage of the menstrual cycle shortened the exposed women's menstrual cycles, while compounds taken from later in the cycle lengthened the exposed women's menstrual cycles. This complex signaling via airborne chemicals is common in lower forms of animals; however, this is the first scientific study proving the signaling in humans.

Top euphemisms for menstruation.
1) Ridin' the cotton pony.
2) Checking into the Red Roof Inn
3) Kate Bush-ing
4) Falling to the Communists
5) A visit form Cap'n Bloodsnatch
6) A visit from Aunt Flo
7) Walking along the beach in soft focus
8) Red Skelton dropped by
9) The Red Sea
10) Getting' down with the O.B.
11) It's that time of the month.
    (Modified from *The Onion*, Vol. 37 (23), 2001)

Just how many "monthlies" do we get? This question usually begets a resounding "*Too many!*" from the audience. Of course they are right. By the time a Western woman reaches age 50, she will have experienced approximately 450 lifetime ovulations or episodes of menses—three times that of her great-grandmother and perhaps her grandmother. Your great-grandmother averaged 190 periods in her lifetime. Why? Are we living longer? Did great-grandma die sooner? Did she have all of her children and subsequently succumb to the rigors of child rearing? Is our "period of having periods" longer?

The answer to the first question is yes, we're living longer, but that has nothing to do with the number of periods you or your grandmother experienced. Did great-grandma die sooner? Yes, but she still outlived her ovaries. Even at the turn of the twentieth century the life expectancy of women was over 50 years of age. So, women did not *die* before their ovaries died. The major differences are three-fold. First, women started having periods in their mid-teens, not in their early adolescent years and certainly not starting around age nine as we are seeing today. Second, women had more children. Five, six and seven kids was more the norm than the 1.8 average number today in the U.S. (My brother is the 0.8.) And, most women in the early twentieth century breast-fed each of their children, usually for up to a year or more. Combine all three of those factors and the number of menstrual periods drops precipitously. The young girls living in our world today start their periods earlier, don't

> *The average woman loses about 2 ounces of blood and 17 mg of iron during a normal menstrual period. The average woman who uses tampons will use 11,400 in her lifetime.*

have as many children, and don't breast feed. Now, before you take exception to that last reason, I do realize that women do breast feed in the United States, but the numbers are far less and the length of time is much less than women of past generations.

Sanitary napkins. The precursor to today's sanitary napkin can be attributed to French Army nurses during World War I. They discovered that the cellulose material used for dressing and absorbing blood from wounds also worked well for absorbing menstrual blood. They discarded the cloth pads they had been using for their "monthlies" and began using the cellulose wound dressings for their periods.

After World War I, the Kimberly Clark Corporation, the supplier to the U.S. Army of cellulose bandages, reported an overabundance of the dressings and they were perplexed as to what to do with them. Someone in the corporation reported the French Army Nurses' use of the dressings and the rest is history. Kimberly Clark adopted the idea and the "sanitary pad" became available for commercial use in 1921. Kimberly Clark chose the name "Kotex," as the designation for the first disposable sanitary napkin. "Modess" by Johnson and Johnson, Inc. followed it shortly.

Tampons and dioxin—a link to endometriosis? Are tampons safe?
The most controversial aspect of tampon safety relates to dioxin. Dioxin is a chemical by-product produced when the cotton and rayon used in tampon production, is bleached using chlorine. Chlorine makes the tampon "look" white and clean. However, the by-product, dioxin, has been linked to an increased risk of developing ectopic endometrial tissue in monkeys—a condition referred to as endometriosis. In one study, almost 80 percent of the monkeys exposed to dioxin developed endometriosis. The monkeys exposed to the highest levels of dioxin devel-

oped the most severe endometriosis. Now remember, this study was done in monkeys, not humans and the verdict is still out as far as humans are concerned.

Dr. Andrew Weil's May 2003 newsletter, *Self-Healing,* quotes the FDA (Food and Drug Administration) and says that tampons contain only a trace of dioxin, which are not a concern. He goes on to say that there is currently no evidence to support any link between tampons and chronic illness such as endometriosis as well as cancer.

Historical Highlights

In 1936, a Denver physician, Dr. Earle Haas, invented a cardboard tube of compressed cotton with a little string inside. Tampons hit the market amid much controversy, ridicule, and scorn, with the misconception that inserting the tampon would "deflower" all of the virgins of the world.

(Endometriosis Association, 8585 N. 76th Place, Milwaukee, WI. 53223. **For dioxin-free products call Terra Femme @ 800-755-0212 or Organic Essentials @ 800-765-4491.)

Endometriosis and other conditions. A survey of 3,600 women with endometriosis found that they were 100 times more likely to experience chronic fatigue syndrome, seven times more likely to have hypothyroidism, twice as likely to experience fibromyalgia, and have higher rates of lupus, rheumatoid arthritis, and multiple sclerosis. Keep this in mind when women with endometriosis have other nonspecific complaints. (*Human Reproduction,* October 2002)

An especially high risk of endometriosis and autoimmune disorders occurs in women with red hair. Keep that in mind when trying to make the diagnosis. (*Fertility and Sterility,* February 1996.)

Rely tampons, super absorbency, and Toxic Shock Syndrome. The Tampax company was the reigning tampon titan through the 1960s; however, by the early 1970s the competition was heating up. All of the big companies wanted a piece of the action. Proctor and Gamble, Playtex, Kimberly-Clark, and Johnson and Johnson all decided to throw their products on the market. So, how could they trump the competition? What would make their product special?

Proctor and Gamble won the competition and came out with the first super-dooper, super absorbent, super polyester "plug." In fact it was basically the size of a telephone poll covered with polyester. The Proctor and Gamble tampon made its debut as the "Rely" tampon in 1979. As in, you can "Rely" on our tampon to not leak and cause those embarrassing moments in your white pedal-pushers at the Labor Day picnic. The Rely tampon could absorb nearly *20* times its own body weight in fluids. Oh my. It could absorb your menstrual period plus everyone else's within a five-mile radius.

In fact, it was so absorbent that all vaginal fluids would be absorbed including the protective vaginal mucus. Women could insert the tampon without a hassle, but removing it was the problem. The early 1980s experienced a flood of women arriving at doctor's offices and emergency rooms for tampon removals.

By the early 1980s the CDC was receiving reports of a sudden surge in Toxic Shock Syndrome (TSS) from the state of Wisconsin. All but one of the cases happened to be menstruating females. Between 1975 and 1980, 95 percent of the women contracting TSS were menstruating at the time. Seventy-one percent were using Rely tampons. If Rely wasn't the tampon implicated specifically, the women were using other brands of super-dooper absorbent tampons. The CDC suggested that super absorbent tampons, when left inside the vagina for longer than six hours at a time, provided a perfect growth environment for *Staphylococcus aureus*, the bacterial cause of what became known as *Staphylococcal* Toxic Shock Syndrome.

The dreaded "laryngopathia premenstrualis." Vocal changes in the immediate premenstrual period are associated with fluctuations in estrogen and progesterone. This condition, "laryngopathia premenstrualis" is believed to be rather common, and is caused by anatomic and physiologic alterations in the vocal cords specifically due to the drop in estrogen. The voice changes are characterized by decreased vocal efficiency, loss of the high-pitched notes in the singing voice, vocal fatigue, hoarseness, and some muffling of the voice.

Drugs that inhibit ovulation, such as oral contraceptives, have been shown to alleviate some of these symptoms. However, oral contraceptives may also alter voice range and character in about 5 percent of the women who take them. This could be a particularly bothersome side effect for female vocalists or opera singers who must consistently hit those high notes. The estrogen drop at menopause can cause the same symptoms, however, estrogen replacement therapy will help to maintain vocal quality in postmenopausal females. (*Hospital Medicine*, March 1997)

One *BIG* reason for oral contraceptive failure. Overweight women who are on oral contraceptives have 60 percent more unintended pregnancies because of much lower serum levels of their oral contraceptive hormones. Their larger size doesn't take into account the amount of hormones needed to suppress ovulation. The take home message from this study is obvious— women who are overweight need to take higher doses of oral contraceptives in order to achieve effective ovulation-suppressing levels of hormones in their tissues—at least 35 mcg of ethinyl estradiol (the estrogen component) per pill. (*American Family Physician* 2002; 66:852)

Another *big* reason for oral contraceptive failure. St. John's Wort, the so-called "herbal Prozac" interacts with numerous prescription drugs including combined oral contraceptives. (A combined oral contraceptive is an estrogen-progestin combination.) St. John's Wort has been shown to reduce the effectiveness of combined oral contraceptives by up to 50 percent. You'll *think* depressed, when you find out you're pregnant! Bottom line: If you're depressed and on combined oral contraceptives, steer clear of "herbal Prozac" and go with the real thing—-prescription antidepressants.

And yet a third big reason for oral contraceptive failure. It doesn't take a Ph.D. from MIT to figure out this one—forgetting to take your oral contraceptive can get you into *big* trouble. Today's oral contraceptives for normal weight girls contain 20- to

> *It take many nails to build crib, only one screw to fill it.*
> —Old Chinese proverb to remind young women to use contraceptive methods as directed.

25-micrograms of estrogen per pill. This is just enough to stop ovulation but not enough to stop the production of a mature egg. So, the egg is waiting in the wings for you to forget your pill and as soon as you do, she bursts out of that ovary and careens down the Fallopian tube lookin' for love. If there is a sperm within a 300-mile radius it will find the lovelorn egg.

The oral contraceptives of yesteryear. Contrast today's oral contraceptives with the first oral contraceptives to hit the market. The first birth control pills in the late 1950's and early 1960s contained enough estrogen to stop an elephant from ovulating. In fact, if you missed two or three pills you didn't have to worry about a surprise pregnancy. And, when you stopped the oral contraceptives in order to conceive, it usually took at least six months to start ovulating again. The first birth control pills contained an average of 80 micrograms of estrogen per pill.

Breast cancer risk and alcohol. The benefits of alcohol on the cardiovascular system may or may not outweigh the risks for breast cancer. Accumulating evidence suggests that alcohol consumption increases the risk for breast cancer, presumably because of its effect on estrogen levels and its potentially negative effects on DNA repair and the immune system.

A woman's breast cancer risk increases by 9 percent for every 10 grams of alcohol consumed on a daily basis. (A 4-ounce glass of wine contains approximately 11 grams of alcohol, a 12-ounce beer contains 13 grams of alcohol, and a shot [1 ounce] of liquor contains 15 grams of alcohol). In a study published in the *American Journal of Epidemiology*, researchers found breast cancer risk elevations of 11 percent, 24 percent, and 38 percent for females consuming one, two, or three drinks per day, respectively.

Most experts currently recommend no more than one drink a day on three to four days of the week. Women on hormone replacement therapy (HRT) should be aware of another study in the *Journal of the American Medical Association* that suggests alcohol has a potentially dramatic effect on estrogen levels. Estrogen levels nearly doubled when women on HRT drank the equivalent of just one-half of a glass of wine. At alcohol levels associated with the equivalent of three glasses of wine, women's estrogen levels rose a whopping 327 percent. (No, that is *not* a typo…*327 percent is correct* in women on HRT.)

What's the good news, you might ask? In a recent study published in the April 2000 *American Journal of Epidemiology*, women aged 75 and older reported that drinking one to three glasses of wine every day (or one to three beers/one to three ounces of liquor) may increase bone mass by increasing estrogen levels. Estrogen has a positive effect on the bone-building cells known as the osteoblasts. In addition, since alcohol (in moderation, of course) increases estrogen, it has a secondary effect of boosting mental acuity.

Antiperspirants *do not* cause breast cancer. This definitive study can finally throw this baby out with the bath water. Emails have been circulating for a few years screaming about the hazards of antiperspirants and deodorants and how they increase the risk of breast cancer. The theory was that they block the release of toxins and carcinogens from being excreted from the armpits, and that these toxins accumulate in the lymph system where they trigger breast cancer, and *blah,blah,blah.* Well, dear readers, this is another Internet hoax so please let your friends, colleagues, and even enemies know that they should commence wearing deodorant again. It will do wonders for their social life and for the comfort of all those in the surrounding environs. (*Journal of the National Cancer Institute,* October 16, 2002)

Breast cancer—historical perspectives. How long breast cancer has been killing women cannot be directly ascertained; however, it can be traced back farther than any other cancer. The earliest recorded cases of tumors or ulcers of the breasts were recorded in the Egyptian Pyramid Age (circa 3000-2500 BC) with the following commentary:

"Bulging tumors of the breast mean the existence of swellings on the breast, large, spreading and hard; touching them is like touching a ball of wrappings or they may be compared to the unripe hemat-fruit which is hard and cool to the touch like swellings on the breast."

The writings of Herodutus, a historian who lived just prior to Hippocrates, describe the experiences of Atossa, daughter of Cyrus and wife of Darius. She was described as having a tumor of the breast, which, after a time, ulcerated and spread. So long as it was small, she concealed it and told no one about it, but when it commenced to grow and give her trouble she sent for the famous physician Democedes (Greece, 525 BC). He apparently cured her; however, no mention of his therapeutic method was made.

It frequently comes as a startling revelation to find that many of our cherished clinical observations of the present day have been so clearly described in ancient scholarly works. Hippocrates (400 BC) made a prophetic statement concerning the contraindications of surgery for deep-seated breast cancers. He stated:

"It is better to omit treatment altogether; for if treated, the patients soon die whereas if left alone, they may last a long time."

Now that statement would send the present day internist or surgeon into a tailspin.

Leonides of Alexandria, circa 180 BC, was the first to describe nipple retraction as the most important clinical sign of breast cancer. Unfortunately, it is now known that nipple retraction is a *late* sign of breast cancer, not an early finding.

Aetius of Mesopotamia noted that breast cancer may present as an ulcerated mass, but most often the breast tumor is hard and irregular. He also described it as having extensive roots and as being accompanied by varicose veins. Again, late diagnostic signs appear to be the norm in the days of yesteryear.

The medical treatment of breast cancer included mineral oils, vegetable extracts, and animal wastes. Innumerable psychic and physical agents were used. Caustics were skillfully applied by Egyptians, Romans and Greeks, and were particularly well developed by the Arabian School of Medicine. Once again, Hippocrates added his two cents about the numerous treatment modalities used to treat breast cancer.

"Those diseases that medicines do not cure, are cured by the knife. Those that the knife does not cure are cured by fire. Those that fire does not cure, must be considered incurable."

During the Dark Ages of medicine, surgeons demonstrated a multitude of mutilating treatments—from cauterization and radical surgery to compressing cancers of the breast with a lead plate. By the seventeenth century surgeons began removing enlarged axillary nodes when the breast was radically excised. Exorcism was also used, as were charms and amulets.

The early methods of mastectomy, although rather barbaric and crude to our way of thinking, were surprisingly efficient and probably the result of expediency at a time when speed was of essence in the operating room. Unfortunately the science of anesthesia was by no means advanced so one can only imagine the horrors associated with the pain and mutilating effects of surgery, not to mention the postoperative mortality rate from infection. In order to remove the breast with haste, surgeons passed heavy ligatures horizontally and vertically through the base of the breast. Everyone present in the operating room would grab a handful of the sutures and traction was applied with equal force in all directions resulting in the swift amputation of the breast. Bleeding from the operative area was quickly seared with a hot iron. *Ouch.*

Some things change, some things never change. Women have always taken great pride in their breasts and continue to do so. From the stylish days of décolleté dresses to the present day of breast cosmetic surgery, vanity has always been the so-called death trap of reason in the struggle toward the early diagnosis and treatment of breast cancer.

Cosmetic considerations and false modesty have hindered the early diagnosis and timely treatment of breast cancer from the days of the Egyptian pharaohs to the present day.

With the modern era of medicine came the first real discussion of the facts and figures concerning prognosis and survival. Varying statistics were reported—one group reported 60 cases of breast cancer treated surgically with only four free of disease after two years. Another reported 118 cases with no cures. It appeared as if cancer of the breast was associated with a high mortality rate. During this period, prevailing pessimism indicated that the most one could ever expect from an operation for breast cancer was that the patient might die a little less miserably.

> *Up until the seventeenth century it was a customary and respectful form of salutation to touch the breasts in a warm, friendly greeting.*

Surgical treatment and prognosis for breast cancer improved considerably with Dr. Halsted's introduction of the radical mastectomy in the early twentieth century. Dr. Halsted believed that the aggressive local management of the primary tumor with extensive removal of surrounding lymph nodes and underlying pectoral muscles would control the spread of disease. In the 1970s, Fisher broke ranks with the traditional Halstedian approach to radical mastectomy. He disagreed with the theory that radical surgery would control the disease. He argued that microscopic metastases were already present at initial diagnosis in patients who would later manifest widespread metastatic disease and thus local aggressive surgical procedures such as radical mastectomy were unnecessary. His approach shifted therapeutic emphasis to earlier systemic therapy with minimal local surgical treatment. This treatment strategy has replaced Dr. Halsted's strategy. Breast-conserving surgery and adjuvant systemic therapies are offered to most patients with early breast cancer today.

Breast compression and mammograms. Compression of the breasts for mammography requires 25-40 pounds of pressure. Any woman who has had a "mammiogram" can attest to this pressure as the tech continues to "wind it up a notch." For those of us with large breasts it continues to be a source of amazement as to just how flat the mammogram technician can make them. Pancake flatness comes to mind immediately as she continues increase the pressure. One can't help but imagine best friends without large, pendulous breasts and how their breasts fit between the two hard plastic plates.

Breast size. Some women are just never satisfied with their breast size. The late Eve Valois of France had 22 breast enlargements during her lifetime. The final size and weight were: 71 inches with a 54G brassiere and their combined weight was 26 pounds. (*Guinness Book of World Records*, 2003)

Breast cancer risk factors. Do factors in the womb influence the development of breast cancer? This is referred to as fetal or prenatal programming and it appears if certain circumstances in utero and possibly immediately after birth may play a role in breast cancer develop-

Historical Highlights

Dr. William Stewart Halsted (1852-1922) was a Professor of Surgery at the Johns Hopkins University in Baltimore, Maryland. He is credited with performing the first resection of cancer of the ampulla of Vater, and he later introduced the use of rubber gloves into the surgical setting. In fact, when Dr. Halsted introduced rubber gloves into the operating suite, he did so to protect the hands of his chief operating room nurse (whom he later married). Nudge, nudge, wink, wink. One of his students subsequently suggested the use of the gloves by the surgeons as well, since the gloves could be sterilized and re-used. He was first to describe the Halsted procedure for treating breast cancer, during which the entire breast as well as the pectoralis major and minor and the lymphatic structures of the axilla are also removed. In 1894 when he first performed this procedure, it was described as a life-saving operation. Today this "radical mastectomy" or Halsted procedure has been almost exclusively replaced with less invasive, breast-conserving surgeries such as the modified mastectomy, the quadrantectomy, and the lumpectomy.

ment in later years. Three conditions are associated with future breast cancer risk. These include birth weight, toxemia during the third trimester of pregnancy, and jaundice in early postnatal life.

Researchers from Uppsala University in Sweden reported that women who had weighed eight pounds or more at birth had a 30 percent greater risk of breast cancer later in life. Being scrawny at birth offers some protection. The risk of breast cancer for women who weighed 5.5 pounds or less at birth was less than half the risk faced by women who had tipped the delivery scales at greater than eight pounds.

In addition, statistical analysis has revealed a sharply reduced risk of breast cancer among women whose mothers had developed pregnancy-induced hypertension. Such women showed nearly a 60 percent *reduction* in breast cancer risk.

Finally, women who had jaundice as newborns later had an increased risk of breast cancer. A few studies have found that jaundiced babies have high concentrations of estrogen in their bloodstream, hence the increased risk of breast cancer.

The importance of breast self exams (BSE) revisited for the ump-teenth time. It looks like the verdict is finally in and the verdict is: breast self-examination is out, kind of. The study, supported by the National Institutes of Health, was conducted jointly by Chinese researchers and American researchers from the Fred Hutchinson Cancer Research Center in Seattle. Approximately 133,000 women working in Chinese factories were given intensive BSE instruction with reinforcement sessions. The control group, also consisting of approximately 133,000 women, received no BSE instruction. Neither group had the luxury of annual mammograms.

After ten years of follow-up, the number of breast cancer related deaths were virtually identical in the two groups (135 in the BSE group and 131 in the control group). Interesting, eh? The overall death rate was *higher* in the BSE group compared to the control group. Of course this wasn't statistically significant, however, the numbers were still annoying.

> *From the biological point of view, the story of fetal programming shows clearly that for the health of our society, women's health is more important than men's.*
> —(Peter Nathanielsz, *Prenatal Prescription*, 2001.)

Bottom line #1. Results from this huge trial suggest that large-scale efforts to teach BSE are unlikely to lead to a reduction in breast cancer deaths. What this study doesn't answer is whether or not BSE combined with clinical examinations or mammography might result in different findings. The conclusion of the authors is summarized in an editorial entitled "Routinely teaching breast self-examination is dead: What does this mean?" (*J Natl Cancer Inst* 2002 Oct 2; 94:1420-1)

Bottom line #2. The findings don't mean that women should stop breast self-exams. However, we should not have unrealistic expectations about their value. When breast lumps are found early, and if malignant, and if treatment is started early, the prognosis improves. In addition, breast exams give a woman a sense of control over their own breast destiny. So, for now, we are still recommending self breast exams. Keep them up.

Breast-feeding. Breast milk has been recommended for the treatment of cataracts, burns, eczema and "expelling noxious excrements in the belly of a man." The wet nurses of ancient Egypt were held in highest esteem. A royal wet nurse was invited to royal births, royal weddings, and royal funerals. The children of the royal wet nurse were considered "milk kin" to the king.

As far back as the seventh century B.C. there are reports of the King of Assyria being artificially being fed with cow's milk.

A collection of writings from India, the Sushruta Samhita (2200-2400 years old) prescribed that various herbs, extracts, honey and butter be given to the newborn before breast-feeding was started. Delaying breast-feeding was common. Soreanus, (pronounced sore'eh nus) a Greek M.D. in the second century A.D.) taught that nothing should be given for the first two days and then animal milk for three weeks. The practice of prelacteal feeding still occurs widely in India but with a well-known increased risk of infection in the newborn.

The Milky Way. The breast milk of the Greek goddess Hera was said to confer infinite life on those who drank it. When Zeus sought divinity for his son Hercules, born of an adulterous affair with the mortal Alcmena, he sneaked the infant into the bedroom of his sleeping wife Hera, and put Hercules to her breast for a taste of her milk. Hercules sucked so hard that Hera woke, and she shook him off in outrage, spurting milk across the skies—hence, the Milky Way. Fortunately for young Hercules he had swallowed enough of the breast milk to join the ranks of the immortals.

Saint Agattin—the Saint of nursing women. The association of a saint with a disease or clinical conditions was sometimes determined by the manner in which the saint died. St. Agattin was tortured prior to death and part of the torture was cutting her breasts off. For that reason, she has been designated the patron saint of diseases of the breast as well as the patron saint of the nursing woman.

External pelvic massage. The electromechanical vibrator made its debut in the early 1880s and the reason for its debut is rather fascinating. It was developed to perfect and automate a function that doctors had performed for women for many years. The procedure was for the "the relief of physical, emotional and sexual tension through the use of external pelvic massage, culminating in orgasm." External pelvic massage is a fancy way of saying masturbation and in the 1880s women paid handsomely for their physician to perform this procedure in the office.

Physicians documented that this external pelvic massage, also known as vulvar massage, would cure just about any symptoms that the woman might have—including symptoms labeled at the time as "hysterical" and "neurasthenic." Of course, one of the ongoing benefits of this treatment was that the woman would continually return to that specific doctor for her "routine" check-ups, so to speak. Anyway, the invention of the vibrator made this a quick, easy, and clean routine—no fuss no muss, get 'em in, and get 'em out. Sounds like the earliest HMO's. Prevention is the best medicine.

Vibrators were marketed as home appliances and they were among the first "home appliances" to use electricity. In fact, vibrators were the fifth household appliance to use electricity with the sewing machine, fan, teakettle and toaster as the first four. The vacuum cleaner and the electric iron were not among the first priorities for use with electricity.

By the turn of the century there were over 20 models of vibrators available to choose from. There were vibrators that played music, vibrators that hung from the ceiling, vibrators that were attached to "jolting chairs," vibratory forks, and floor models on wheels. Some vibrators were faster than the speed of light while

Historical Highlight

The 1899 *Merck Manual*, a reference guide for physicians, lists external pelvic massage, or vulvar massage, as the treatment for hysteria.

def'i·ni'tions

Clitoris is derived from the Greek term, *kleitoris* and is said to be derived from *kleis*, "a door latch," the clitoris being likened to a "latch" on the vagina.

Hymen. From the Greek *hymen* meaning a skin or membrane. The Greek word was used for all sorts of membranes, including the membrane around the heart known as the pericardium and the membrane around the abdominal cavity referred to as the peritoneum. After a period of time, Hymen became the name of the God of Marriage, a sort of overgrown Cupid. It was not until the sixteenth century that "hymen" was restricted to denote the vaginal or virginal membrane.

Hysterectomy. Derived from the combination of the Greek word *hystera*, the womb or uterus, and *tome*, a cutting. To the Greeks, *hysterikos* meant a "suffering in the womb." As far back as Plato's era the uterus was described as becoming "indignant, dissatisfied, and ill-tempered and it caused a general disturbance of the body until it became pregnant." This teaching gave rise to the age-old tendency to attribute various abnormal manifestations to specific body organs. Emotional instability, thought to be more characteristic of females, was blamed on the uterus. From this anatomic designation we use the terms hysteria and hysterical. Female "hysteria" encompassed a varied assortment of ailments including lassitude, irritability, depression, confusion, palpitations, insomnia, headaches, forgetfulness, spasms, stomach upsets, writing cramps, weepiness and even ticklishness.

So, what we're saying here is that in the old days when we *didn't* become pregnant we would become hysterical and have all sorts of spectacular symptoms attributed to our "barren womb." Fast forward to modern times and the scenario changes ever so slightly—when we *do* get pregnant we become hysterical and have all sorts of spectacular symptoms attributed to our "blossoming womb." Once we have finished our child-bearing years we become hysterically happy when they *remove* the cause of our hysteria. In fact, it would be nice if our uterus could just fall out after our last child. A pre-programmed drop-out of the uterus after the birth of little Petunia. Out comes Petunia, out comes the placenta, and plop! Out comes the uterus. If this scenario were to exist, we wouldn't have all of the problems attributed to postmenopausal progesterone therapy (the "PRO" in the PREMPRO, for example.)

others had rpms (rotations per minute) of less than 1,000. Prices ranged from 15 bucks for the hand-held do-it-yourself model to what historian Dr. Rachel Maines called the "Cadillac" of vibrators. This mega-machine was known as the Chattanooga and it retailed at a whopping $200 in 1904—and, you even had to pay for the shipping costs.

We've come a long way baby. The British National Health Service has begun prescribing vibrators to women suffering from a lack of desire. This makes one wonder what's so bad about having a National Health Service if this is one of the services provided, "free of charge" so to speak.

Caesarian section is the procedure whereby an infant is removed from the uterus by incising the anterior abdominal wall of the mother. In ancient times it was regularly undertaken when a childbearing woman died close to delivery. Julius Caesar was presumably born via the abdominal wall incision, hence the eponym.

Estrogen and memory. A Yale University study used magnetic resonance imaging to measure brain activity in women given 1.25 mg of estrogen per day for 21 days compared to women receiving placebo. After a "washout" (no treatment) period of 14 days, the women were switched to the opposite treatment for another 21 days. During both phases of the trial (on-estrogen and off-estrogen), the women were asked to perform verbal and non-verbal tasks during an MRI imaging session. The tasks were designed to test short-term or "working" memory such as the name of the person you just met at a party three minutes ago.

The results of the study were as follows: During estrogen treatment, the women showed significant alterations in brain activity, especially in the areas of the brain associated with short-term memory. In fact, estrogen appeared to

def'i·ni'tions

The word **"hussy"** in the sixteenth century was perfectly respectable; it meant simply a housewife, derived from the short form of the Old English *huswif*. Only a century later, the word had come to mean a bold and shameless woman.

reinstate brain activation patterns associated with younger, but not older, people as they perform memory tasks. This study provides the first visual evidence that estrogen can alter brain circuitry, or organization. (*JAMA*, June 1999)

def'i·ni'tions

Lady. The literal meaning of "lady"—in its Old English form "hlāēfdīge" (through the Middle English "lafdi, ladi")—is "loaf-kneader."
(Asimov)

Kegel exercises for a bigger, better orgasm. Now this is one exercise you might just want to partake in daily. The pubococcygeal (PC) muscle group, which supports the pelvic floor, is the one that spasms when you have an orgasm. If it's in good shape, more blood will flow to the pelvic area during arousal and the PC muscle will contract more strongly, making orgasms last longer and feel more intense. Kegel exercises are a simple way to strengthen PC muscles. To do the Kegel exercise, squeeze the muscle you use to voluntarily hold back your urine. Hold for two seconds and then release. Repeat 20 times, three times a day. You can actually do this anywhere and at anytime. You don't need to go to the gym; you don't need to lie on a floor mat. You can drive to the store and while you're at a stoplight, just *tighten up*. A few times at the stoplight, a few times before you get out of the car, a couple of times going around the block and before you know it, you will have performed 60 Kegel's throughout the day. While you're thinking about it, go ahead; contract those muscles, two, three, four…and again, two, three, four.

Sex and the sacral stimulator. Dr. Stuart Meloy of London has found that by stimulating the third sacral nerve in female subjects, he could induce an orgasm every time. Dr. Meloy has created a device about the size of a cigarette pack that can be implanted into the buttocks and operated by remote control. Could the mass marketing of this device make the male species completely obsolete? Hmmmm.

Orgasm nasal spray? Just one or two snorts per nostril, wait one to two minutes, and voilá! The September 1994 *British Medical Journal* reported on an unexpected benefit received by an Australian woman who administered the hormone oxytocin nasally to assist her with the milk-letdown response and breast-feeding. After receiving two snorts of the oxytocin spray she was so distracted by its pleasurable effects (heightened arousal followed by frantic sex and multiple, intensified orgasms) that she had a difficult time concentrating on breast-feeding.

Before you rush out to your personal OB-GYN physician for a prescription of oxytocin nasal spray, you also need to know that our Australian friend was also on a progesterone-containing birth control pill, levonorgestrel. Once she stopped the oral contraceptive, her sex drive returned to normal, even though she remained on the oxytocin. Researchers speculated that it was the combination of the birth control pill *and* the oxytocin that gave her the extra zip in her doo-dah.

Herbal Viagra for women? In a Stanford study, 77 women took the herbal product *ArginMax for Women,* a blend of L-arginine, herbs, vitamins and minerals. Of the 77 women, 74 percent reported improved sexual satisfaction (desire, frequency, vaginal dryness and sensation) compared to 37 percent in the placebo group.

Spontaneous orgasms in the shopping mall. Well, this young woman with recurrent depression did not have a sacral stimulator but she does have a story to tell. After seeing her physician for her depression, she was prescribed sertraline (Zoloft) 100 mg/day. After taking Zoloft for approximately four weeks, she returned to her physician with complaints of sexual dysfunction. In other words, she was happy but she had absolutely no interest in her new husband of only two years. The physician, realizing that sexual dysfunction is a known side effect of this particular drug and the class of drugs it belongs to (known as the SSRIs or selective serotonin reuptake inhibitors) decided to remedy this "emergency" situation. He prescribed an additional drug, known as buproprion (Wellbutrin), 75 mg/day to treat the sexual dysfunction caused by the Zoloft. She reported continued improvement in sexual function over the next four weeks.

After six weeks on both drugs, she was in the midst of a shopping frenzy when she experienced a spontaneous orgasm in the shopping mall. Upon questioning, she stated that she had mixed feelings about the spontaneous orgasm in a public venue. Hmmm. One would hope so. Anyway, she stated that she found the experience quite pleasurable; however,

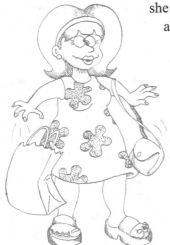

© Ashley Long

she did not feel as if it was socially acceptable in that specific location. She discontinued the Wellbutrin on her own after the experience. Unfortunately the side effect of sexual dysfunction returned. A week later she started back on the Wellbutrin, same dose as before, and the socially unacceptable but personally satisfying side effect returned.

P.S. Since this single case study was reported in *Biological Psychiatry* 40(11); 1996, Wellbutrin (buproprion) has been used to counteract the side effect of sexual dysfunction in patients taking Zoloft (sertraline) and the other SSRIs such as Paxil (paroxetine), Prozac (fluoxetine), and Celexa (citalopram). Most recipients will find that the rare side effect of spontaneous orgasms may be a welcome one.

Pap smears. The average sexually active American woman has endured the annual ritual of having a Pap smear. "Pap" is an abbreviated term for George Papanicolaou, the physician who discovered the procedure. Without going into all of the details of the actual procedure, suffice it to say that the end result is the microscopic examination of cells removed from the outer layer of the cervix as well as the cells removed from a swab of the endocervical canal. When the cytologist (the individual trained to examine the cytos, or cells) peers into the microscope, the cells stare back. The cells are described according to various sizes, shapes, and amounts. Of course, the goal is to have a completely normal-appearing Pap smear with all of the cells smiling sweetly back at the cytologist. So, make sure that a Pap smear is part of your routine gynecological exam, especially if you are sexually active.

Lose a tooth for every child—gum disease during pregnancy. Nearly all pregnant women develop some signs of gum disease due to the hormonal changes associated with pregnancy. Swelling, bleeding, and small foci of infections may develop. Prevention is the best medicine. In other words—don't get pregnant. But if you must, make sure you see your dentist prior to pregnancy, during pregnancy, and perform the usual dental rituals—brush after every meal (or at least twice a day) and floss daily.

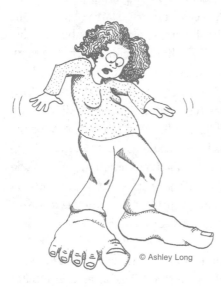

© Ashley Long

Why women's feet grow during pregnancy. At last, here is the answer as to why the feet enlarge during pregnancy. The hormone, relaxin, is produced during the first trimester of pregnancy and continues to be produced throughout. The major function of relaxin is to loosen the tough band of connective tissue fibers inside the cervix and vagina to allow for easy passage of the fetus. Relaxin also relaxes the foot's spring ligament, the one that binds together the bones in the arch of the foot. This newly stretched ligament allows the foot to flatten and spread under the increasing weight of the body. Other changes such as fluid retention, weight gain, and the ducklike gait of pregnancy place stress on parts of the feet that usually don't bear the brunt of the weight. In order to reduce the risk of big feet during pregnancy, one should avoid gaining too much weight and one should wear supportive shoes during the entire nine months. To reverse the big foot problem, lose weight after delivery, and take up a walking program to squeeze fluid out of the tissues of the feet and to help strengthen the muscles around the spring ligament.

Size nine (or any size) high-heeled pumps. For those of you who love high-heels, you might as well

If high heels were so wonderful, men would still be wearing them.
—Sue Grafton

make an appointment with your friendly orthopedist, podiatrist, or chiropractor. Wearing high-heels on a daily basis can lead to extreme curvature of the spine, lower back pain, permanent shortening of the Achilles tendon, and enlarged, displaced calf muscles. Not only that, but you will also walk funny. Feet clad in high-heeled shoes have a difficult time initiating locomotion. Normally the foot propels the leg by opening the angle between the toe and the bottom of the leg. With high-heels, the angle is already open, therefore, it's hard to get-a-goin'; hence, you will have a bit of difficulty walking.

The saga of the perilous pumps—continued. Women have about 90 percent of the 795,000 annual surgeries for bunions, hammertoes, neuromas, and bunionettes. The American Orthopedic Foot and Ankle Society explains the reason: A 3-inch heel creates seven times as much stress on the forefoot as a 1-inch heel. So, the higher the pump, the quicker you'll be in the surgical suite.

Historical Highlights

Many cultures originally used cultivated grains to measure short distances—in particular, the barleycorn had a seed of surprisingly consistent length. Three barleycorns placed end-to-end equaled exactly one inch. This led to the landmark decision by King Edward II of England. He decreed in 1324 that 36 barleycorns would equal one foot, and the rest is history. One more foot fact—the difference between shoe sizes is exactly one barleycorn or one-third of an inch. In other words, a size seven is one-third of an inch longer than a size six. A size nine is exactly one inch longer than a size six. So, how many barleycorns did your feet enlarge during pregnancy?

High-heels and the level of education. Can you tell a women's level of education just by looking at her heels? A survey by the American Orthopedic Foot and Ankle Society of 531 women who work outside the home revealed that the higher a woman's education level, the lower the heels of her shoes. Fifty-eight percent of the women with more than four years of college wear flats (shoes with heels lower than one inch), compared with 46 percent of women with a 4-year degree, 40 percent of the women with less than four years of college, and 37 percent of women who have a high school education or less. (*American Family Physician* 1999; 59(8):2008)

Toxic effects of cigarette smoking on the ovary. A study in the January 1999 issue of *Obstetrics and Gynecology* found that women who smoked 20 or more cigarettes per day were four times more likely to have shorter menstrual cycles than women who did not smoke. Smoking 10 cigarettes per day was associated with more variable cycle lengths and bleeding patterns. In addition, women who had at least 10 pack-years of exposure were more likely to have short cycles, anovulation (lack of egg production), and short luteal phases.

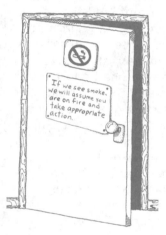

The cigarette smoking bottom line. Cigarette smoking shortens the menstrual cycle in a dose-dependent manner. The follicular phase of the cycle appears to receive the brunt of the damage, suggesting direct toxicity of tobacco by-products on oocyte (egg) development. This may be the reason that smokers have lower estrogen levels, increased problems with fertility and higher miscarriage rates than non-smokers.

Droopy eyelids and premature menopause. Now here's a connection that could only have been made through the extensive painstaking research into the genome project. Perhaps it's not one of the most clinically useful bits of information discerned from years of slaving over DNA splicing, but it certainly could be useful to a select few women—those born with droopy eyelids to name one.

Droopy eyelids in newborns appear to be related to the early onset of menopause decades later. Both conditions, when they occur together, are considered to be the result of a genetic mutation. The FOXL2 gene, newly identified via the genome project, is required not only for normal eyelid development in the fetus, but it is also needed to form a full comple-

Historical Highlights

From the Mount Hope Institute of the Insane (1849), Dr. W. H. Stokes says, in respect to moral sanity: "Another fertile source of this species of derangement appears to be an undue indulgence in the perusal of the numerous works of fiction, with which the press is so prolific of late years, and which are sown widely over the land, with the effect of vitiating the taste and corrupting the morals of the young. Parents cannot too cautiously guard their young daughters against this pernicious practice."

In 1873, Edward H. Clarke, an esteemed Harvard physician, claimed to have discovered the reason for "female sterility." The cause, he wrote, was the education of women, which diverted energy from the reproductivemachinery to the brain, resulting in women with "monstrous brains and puny bodies." It took another 50 years for esteemed researchers to reluctantly admit that low sperm counts in men were also a significant cause of sterility.

ment of eggs in the ovaries before birth. (Remember you get *all* the eggs you're ever going to get prior to birth, ladies. See Chapter 3.)

If there happens to be a mutation in the FOXL2 gene, babies may be born with blepharophimosis (bleh-faro-fi-mo'-sis), or droopy eyelids, and along with those "bedroom" eyes, she may also run through her entire complement of eggs by the age of 30 to 35—a full 10 to 15 years prior to the usual onset of menopause.

This discovery may shed light on certain aspects of aging, which may be driven by genetic processes that begin in the womb, soon after conception. Up

For sale by owner: Complete set of Encyclopedia Brittanica, 45 volumes. Excellent condition, $1,000 or best offer. No longer needed. Got married last weekend. Wife knows everything.
—Ad in New York Post

to 30 percent of women with premature ovarian failure have at least one female relative with blepharophimosis, strongly suggesting that many cases might just be inherited. FOXL2 is a transcription factor, meaning it stimulates other genes to turn "on" or turn "off" in the eyelids and the ovaries at the appropriate time. A mutation in one or two copies of this gene disrupts this process, so genes that would normally be activated by FOXL2 remain dormant, inactive genes might be inappropriately activated or both.

> *I have so little sex appeal that my gynecologist calls me 'sir'.*
> –Joan Rivers

The implications of this research breakthrough are clear. The next time you run into a woman with droopy eyelids you may want to inquire as to the viability of her reproductive status. Or not.

Ovulation and physical attraction. The June 24, 1999 issue of *Nature* published an interesting bit of research on the physical characteristics of male attractiveness during certain phases of the menstrual cycle. When conception chances were the highest at ovulation, women seeking a short-term relationship preferred the "masculinized" look of a squarer jaw and wider face, which may indicate good health. During the other phases of the menstrual cycle, women favored more feminized faces, traits that would make a man a good father and husband. These traits would be trustworthiness and faithfulness versus the more masculine look that would make a great one-night stand.

Big hips and physical attraction. While women are looking at prominent chins and big cheekbones, men are checking out the size of women's hips. When a woman's hips are one-third larger than their waist, they are more physically attractive to men. This feature screams out "I am capable of bearing many, many babies with these big ol' hips. Love me."

The gene for big butts. Scientists have found the gene that gives some sheep unusually big, muscular bottoms and have named this gene *callipyge* (from the Greek for "shapely buttocks"). This gene converts food into muscle 30 percent more efficiently than usual. How annoying is that? However, on a brighter side, discovery of this gene may lead to better insight into fat metabolism and muscle formation. (*Genome Research*, October 2002)

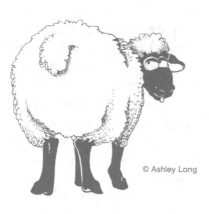

© Ashley Long

Fingers and female fertility. If your index finger is longer than your ring finger, you may be more fertile than your shorter-digited best friend. Researchers from the University of Liverpool in England recently discovered that the gene that controls sex organ growth and differentiation is also responsible for the formation of the fingers and the toes. The researchers also found that women with longer index fingers had higher levels of reproductive hormones. (*American Health,* February 1999)

The early days of female contraception. In the 1920s and 1930s, Margaret Sanger, the birth control crusader, made a valiant attempt to legitimize diaphragms as a physician-prescribed device to be distributed through clinics and physician's offices for poor

Ovulation. *It takes, on average 72 seconds for the mature egg to be pushed out of the ovary. The fertilized egg remains within the Fallopian tube for approximately three days before it enters the uterus.*

Historical Highlights

For founding a birth control clinic in 1917, Margaret Sanger was jailed for a month in the workhouse. By the way, Margaret Sanger, the birth control pioneer, was one of eleven children.

women. The popularity of diaphragms landed with a thud however, and the sale of over-the-counter-products blossomed. By 1938, over-the-counter contraceptives garnered 85 percent of the market. Over-the-counter products had to be marketed under the guise of being a "feminine hygiene" product. Laws at the time forbade the advertising of contraceptives.

Concerned about pregnancy in your teenage daughter? You may want to get your daughter involved in the world of sports. It appears as if being involved with sports is an extremely effective form of birth control. High school girls who are involved in sports are 80 percent less likely to become pregnant than girls who are not involved in sports. Another added benefit—girls involved in sports are three times more likely to get their high school diplomas than non-participants.

Hot flashes and vaginal dryness? Pull out the old toothbrush and wash those symptoms right down the drain. Yes, there may be a mint-flavored toothpaste containing a little dash of estrogen in the near future. Instead of taking a pill, just a 2-minute brushing will take care of those menopausal symptoms. The estrogen will be absorbed right through the mucous membranes of the cheeks and signal the hypothalamus to turn down the flashes. This is one toothpaste tube that should not be shared with your spouse, however. The estrogen can cross the male mucous membranes just as easily and, if used frequently, it can feminize your husband.

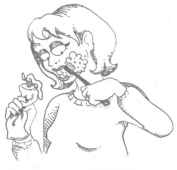

© Ashley Long

> *You should never say anything to a woman that even remotely suggests that you think she's pregnant unless you have received a baby shower announcement.*
> —Anonymous

Hmmmm…nothing worse than your husband wearing a bigger bra than you. His breasts will enlarge, his penis will shrink, his testicles will disappear, and his libido will be kaput.

Liposuction stats. The risk of death from liposuction (now referred to as lipoplasty) was 1 in 5,000 patients in 1998. That risk dropped to 1 in 47,415 from 1998 to 2000. (*Anesthetic Surgery Journal*, March/April 2001)

Sewing machines. The generally accepted start up date for the Industrial Revolution is roughly 1750, but it took a century for development of the first product that specifically lightened women's household tasks. It was Elias Howe's sewing machine.

Stressed out? Rev up the old Singer. If you're feeling out of control, head to your favorite fabric store, purchase a new pattern and fabric, turn on your heel, head home, yank the Singer out of the closet, and put the petal to the metal. In a study commissioned by the American Home Sewing and Craft Association, sewing was found to decrease circulating

> *Last night I discovered a new form of oral contraception. I asked a girl to go to bed with me and she said no.*
> –Woody Allen

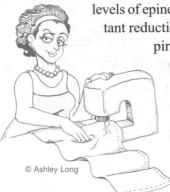
© Ashley Long

levels of epinephrine and norepinephrine with concomitant reductions in heart rate, blood pressure, and respiratory rate. The study actually compared sewing to four other activities—playing cards, painting at an easel, reading a newspaper, and playing a hand-held video game. Sewing beat the competition, hands down.

Sewing machines and masturbation. Robert Taylor, writing in 1905, warned that horseback riding, use of sewing machines, and bicycle riding could all lead to female masturbation, but he also admitted that "in general no great harm is done to the system by the habit." (Maines, RP. *The Technology of Orgasm.* Johns Hopkins University Press, Baltimore, 1999.)

Dorothea Dix, the nineteenth century educator and first superintendent of U.S. Army nurses, recommended as nurses only women who were strong and not-too-good-looking.

Wives and heart disease. The wives of men who have heart disease are also at risk because of the shared lifestyle. The wives share risk factors such as smoking, lack of exercise, unhealthy diet and being overweight. A recent study of 177 men recovering from a heart attack or bypass surgery and their wives showed that the wives could be at an even greater risk. The men had an average cholesterol level of 210, while the women had an average of 226. The couples were slightly overweight on average, and the stress of caring for an ill husband could potentially make the wife's situation much worse.

How often is an egg a lemon? Up to 60 percent of pregnancies end in fetal loss, and most of this loss is believed to occur four to five weeks between conception and

> *Women with high levels of estrogen appear as much as eight years younger than their actual age, while those with low levels of estrogen tend to look older than their actual age.* (U. of Ertlangen-Nurnberg, Germany and U. of Chile, Santiago)

the clinically recognized pregnancy. Swedish obstetricians and geneticists examined the causes of this fetal loss. They studied women between the ages of 25 and 38 who were undergoing laparoscopy as a part of an infertility work-up. During this procedure the researchers aspirated ovarian follicles and examined each follicle under a light microscope. They found that nearly half of all eggs collected had abnormal genetic information. These chromosomally abnormal eggs are most likely responsible for the large number of spontaneous abortions and fetal losses. Corresponding studies on male sperm revealed abnormal genes in only ten percent.

Some notes on fertility. Natural fertility in women peaks at 24 and declines thereafter. A sharp decline is noted after age 37 and 20 percent of U.S. women have their first child after 35. By age 40 to 45 up to 80 percent of the oocytes (eggs) will have chromosomal abnormalities but the uterus remains receptive to implantation. Infertility evaluations should be started after one or more years of unprotected intercourse with no conception or consider an earlier work-up for women over age 35 or those with obvious historical factors suggesting difficulty.

Historical Highlights

"Son of a gun!" In the nineteenth century the British Navy occasionally allowed the spouses of sailors to accompany their husbands to sea. Because the ship's deck had to be kept clear, the only place a woman could give birth aboard ship was behind a canvas shelter placed between the cannons on the gun deck—hence the term, "son of a gun!"

The seahorse. The female seahorse impregnates the male seahorse with about 600 eggs. He then washes his sperm over the eggs and fertilizes the group. About 50 days later the male seahorse begins labor and gives birth to 600 little seahorsies.

© Ashley Long

Weight gain and asthma. Women who gain 50 or more pounds after their eighteenth birthday are five times more likely to develop asthma compared to those with stable weight. The mechanism by which obesity might trigger adult onset asthma is not clear, however, three mechanisms might contribute: 1) a reduction in airflow due to obesity, 2) gastroesophageal reflux triggering bronchospasm, and 3) excess estrogen in adipose tissue. Estrogen has been linked to a higher risk of asthma, and there is a direct correlation between the amount of estrogen in the body and the amount of fat tissue. (*Archives of Internal Medicine*, November 1999)

> *If you want to lose 170 pounds right away, get rid of your husband.*
> —George Burns

Weight gain during pregnancy and breast cancer risk. A report from the *Internal Medicine News* stated that pregnant women who gained as little as three pounds over the recommended 35-pound limit were 40 percent more likely to develop breast cancer after menopause than those who gained only 25 to 30 pounds.

Speaking of weight gain. Women typically gain 4 to 18 pounds per decade as a part of the "aging" process. Bummer.

Are we _still_ speaking about weight gain? Weight gain and heart disease risk. A study in the February 8, 1995 _Journal of the American Medical Association_ suggests that women who gain even a modest amount of weight with aging face an increased risk of heart disease compared to those who manage to keep their weight on an even keel. The findings were surprising:

- Women who gain 11 to 17 pounds over their weight at age 18 run a 25 percent increased risk of heart disease as compared to peers who had gained fewer than 11 pounds.

- Women who gain 17 to 24 pounds showed a 64 percent greater risk.

- Women who gain 44 pounds or more face the most serious threat— a 250 percent greater risk.

The top 10 causes of death in women:
1) Heart disease
2) Cancer
3) Cerebrovascular disease
4) Chronic obstructive pulmonary disease
5) Pneumonia
6) Influenzae
7) Diabetes
8) Accidents and adverse drug effects
9) Alzheimer's disease
10) Nephritis and septicemia

(_American Family Physician_, July 1998; 58(1): 27)

Premarin cream for recurrent nosebleeds. Yes, that's what I said. You mean Premarin _vaginal_ cream? Yes, that's what I said. Vaginal cream will work on any mucous membrane area and it just so happens that in the nasal mucosa, Premarin vaginal cream builds up the tissue and protects the dense capillary system from local trauma (e.g., a finger, fingernail, Q-tip, elbow, tissue, etc.). Apply the Premarin vaginal cream twice a day to the offending nostril for one month. Consider topical estrogen for recurrent nosebleeds that don't respond to the usual treatments. A compounded nasal spray is also available. It contains 0.67

percent of injectable Premarin in normal saline. Administer 1 spray to the offending nostril three times per day.

Estrogen replacement therapy and breast density. Approximately 31 percent of postmenopausal women on continuous estrogen and progesterone therapy may experience a significant increase in breast density as evidenced by changes in the first post-treatment mammogram. It may be prudent to change to a different regimen. Cyclic combinations of hormone therapy and estrogen alone did not cause a change in breast density. Remember that changes in breast density lower the sensitivity and specificity of mammograms. (Sendage F, et al. *Fertility and Sterility* 2001 [September]; 445-50)

An ancient test for virginity. This is a test devised by a rabbi and recorded in the Talmud. His test consisted of seating two women, a virgin and a non-virgin, in turn, on a barrel of wine. The examiner would then smell the breath of each young woman. The breath of the non-virgin smelled of wine, whereas the breath of the virgin did not. It was presumed that the intact hymen prevented the odor of the wine ascending through the body. The test was obviously not based on sound physiological and anatomical principles. The hymen blocks the reproductive tract, not the gastrointestinal tract or the respiratory tract

An ancient test for pregnancy. The ancient Roman physicians measured the neck size daily in women presumed to be pregnant. The test was based on the knowledge that thyroid enlargement occurs in pregnant women due to the increase in metabolism and energy requirements required to maintain the pregnancy. A similar test was used in the United States in colonial times. A girl was considered a virgin if a string, which was stretched from the tip of her nose to the end of her sagittal suture at the point where it joins the lamboidal suture, can then wrap around her neck. If the string cannot reach all the way around, her thyroid is enlarged and she was considered to be "in the family way." Just think of all of the money spent on pregnancy tests, ultrasounds, blood tests, etc., when just a simple ball of string will do.

Gardening and osteoporosis. In a study of 3,000 women over age 50, a University of Arkansas researcher has found that gardening and yard work rank with weight training—ahead of all activities such as swimming and walking—in helping prevent osteoporosis. The highest levels of bone density were found in women who lifted weights or worked in the yard. The weight-bearing motions that go into gardening—such as digging holes, pulling weeds, and pushing a mower—can have significant impact on bone strength.

Ovarian cancer and feminine hygiene products. Several studies over the past decade have correlated the use of feminine hygiene powders and powder-based feminine hygiene sprays with an increased risk of ovarian cancer. A recent study from the University of Washington confirms the past studies with some rather startling conclusions. Researchers compared 322 women with ovarian cancer to 426 women without ovarian cancer. The women with ovarian cancer were 50 percent more likely to have used a powder-based product in their genital area. The increased risk is most likely due to the various chemicals used in the production of scented sprays. If used frequently, the chemicals may wend their way up the Fallopian tubes and lodge in the outer, epithelial layer of the ovary. If the chemicals remain lodged in the outer layer of the ovary for long periods of time, they may act as carcinogens (agents that trigger cancer) and initiate the process of malignant transformation. (Society for Epidemiological Research, "Perineal powder and the Risk of Ovarian Cancer," paper presented in June 1996)

High altitudes and the "saline sloshes." Traveling from low altitudes to high altitudes has an adverse effect on saline breast implants. Dr. James Bachman, a family physician practicing medicine at the Frisco Medical Center in the Colorado Rockies, has seen more than a dozen women complaining of sloshing sounds emanating from their breasts. All of the women were tourists and all of them just happened to have saline breast implants. One of the women complained of a persistent cough so he had the opportunity to order a chest X-ray. The chest X-ray did not determine the cause of the cough, but it did confirm his suspicions concerning the origins of the sloshing noises. Air bubbles were observed in the breasts. Traveling from a low altitude to a high altitude caused air dissolved in the saline to leave the solution. Once the women returned to the low altitudes the sloshing noises disappeared.

Speaking of implants—how about a bit of bovine breast enlargement? In the cutthroat world of bovine beauty contests the size of a cow's udder can be the difference between a blue ribbon and a two-foot trophy and the lowly honorable mention. Before the show, farmers are injecting the udders of their bovine Miss Americas with foam to make them larger. This of course, is cheating, and veterinarians have developed an ultrasound technique for detecting foam implants.

Hair color and employment opportunities. Should you interview for your next job as a redhead, a blonde, or a brunette? Researchers at the University of California, San Marcos, wanted to determine whether hair color and makeup might determine how an employer perceives women seeking professional employment. Researchers asked 136 college students to review the resume and photograph of a 40-year-old blonde-haired female applicant for a job as an accountant. Each student was handed the same resume, but in some photos the blonde hair was altered to red or brown, and in half the photos the woman wore makeup. And the winner is…

As a brunette, the woman was offered a higher salary and rated more capable than she was as a blonde or a redhead. Makeup lowered her competence score and salary, no matter what her hair color was.

This study suggests that societal stereotypes continue to exist and may make a difference in how female job seekers are perceived. This study is particularly interesting in that college students are typically more liberal and open to appearance differences than employers are, and therefore would be less likely to stereotype individuals. (Kyle DJ. Hair color and cosmetic use. *Psyc of Women Quarterly* 1996; Vol. 20)

Aphrodisiac describes a substance said to enhance libido. Aphrodite was the daughter of Zeus and Dione, the goddess of moisture, and was so named because she sprang from the foam of the sea. Aphrodite was the goddess of beauty and sexual love.

Hair products as a hidden source of estrogen. It has been a well-known fact that African American girls start having their periods and enter puberty approximately two to three years earlier than Caucasian girls in the U.S. Many reasons have been proposed, from inactivity to obesity to dietary influences; however, a new reason has appeared in the literature. An article in the *New Scientist* (April 2002) reports that some hair-care products are triggering early adolescence in girls because they contain estrogen. Even though estrogens are supposedly banned in over-the-counter products, some companies continue to market these products, especially to the African-American population. One particular product, B&B Super Gro, is particularly popular with African-American girls. This may explain the puberty onset difference between ethnic groups. Half of the African-American girls in the U.S. begin developing breasts or pubic hair by age eight, as compared to only 15 percent of Caucasian girls.

Ladies lingerie with an alarm. Those Italians think of everything. An Italian inventor recently unveiled a line of microchip-equipped panties that sound a loud alarm when the wearer's bottom is pinched. This line of underwear may soon be coming to a Neimann-Marcus near you.

Historical Highlights

Camels have the distinction of being the first animals to use IUDs. For years, camel drivers would place apricot pits in the uteri of the females so that they would not become pregnant on long caravan trips.

Ancient Egyptians realized that by blocking the passage of seminal fluid from entering the womb, a woman would not become pregnant. So they constructed their own diaphragm that consisted of a lint pad soaked in a mixture of acacia tips and honey. This mixture produces a profound amount of lactic acid, the active ingredient in most contraceptive jellies.

> *The only time a woman wishes she were a year older is when she is expecting a baby.*
> —Anonymous

Migraine headaches— cured by cosmetic surgery? A report in the August 2000 issue of *Plastic and Reconstructive Surgery* provides data concerning patients who had "forehead lifts" for those furrowed brows and subsequently experienced relief from chronic migraine headaches. In a review of 314 patients who had the procedure, researchers found that among the 39 who had suffered migraines prior to surgery, 80 percent experienced an improvement of symptoms or a disappearance of their migraines altogether.

The researchers hypothesize that the surgical removal of the forehead muscle removes a "link" in the chain of events that triggers the migraine. The trigeminal nerve traverses this muscle. Stimulation of the trigeminal nerve releases neurotransmitters that increase nerve sensitivity to pain. Compression of this nerve by the forehead muscle may trigger the onset; therefore removal of the muscle may remove a migraine trigger. (For more information contact Dr. Bahman Guyuron, Department of Plastic and Reconstructive Surgery, Case Western Reserve, Cleveland, Ohio.)

A woman was six months pregnant with her third child, when her three-year-old daughter came into the room just as she was getting ready to hop into the shower. She said, "Mommy, you are getting fat!" The mom replied, "Yes, honey, remember Mommy has a baby growing in her tummy." "I know," the daughter replied, "but what's growing in your butt?"

Cradling the baby in the left arm. Eighty percent of mothers cradle their infants in their left arm. Regardless of race, ethnic group, location, and handedness of the mother, this seems to be a universal trait. In fact, gorillas and chimpanzees frequently cradle their infants and more than 80 percent of the time they cradle on the left side. Many theories have been proposed as to why this left-cradling preference occurs.

One proposed theory is that it leaves mom's right hand free to open doors and baby jars, which sounds feasible until studies revealed that even left-handed women show the same left-cradling preference. The second theory suggests that babies held on the left are soothed by the maternal heartbeat; however, the sound is mostly inaudible in that position.

The third theory, proposed by the University of Liverpool, suggests that the left- cradling dates back six to eight million years. Such long endurance of the habit would suggest that it provides a survival advantage. They speculate that the emotion-laden information is handled by the brain's right side. The right side of the brain has input from the left eye and ear, so that a mother holding her infant on the left side monitors the infant with her left-brain and ear, while using her emotionally savvy right brain. The research also suggests that left-arm cradling and right-brain baby watching results in better bonding between the mother and her infant. This results in a better chance of survival for the little bambino.

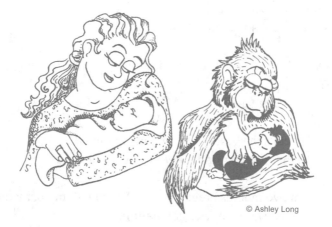

© Ashley Long

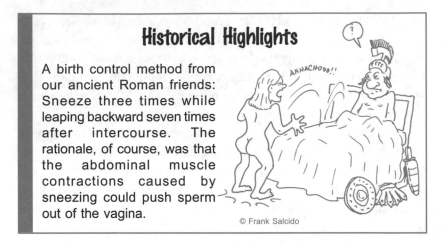

Historical Highlights

A birth control method from our ancient Roman friends: Sneeze three times while leaping backward seven times after intercourse. The rationale, of course, was that the abdominal muscle contractions caused by sneezing could push sperm out of the vagina.

© Frank Salcido

Quiz. This syndrome affects nearly 6 percent of all premenopausal women. It has numerous systemic manifestations including infertility, endometrial cancer, diabetes, and heart disease. In addition, women have male-pattern baldness and an overabundance of coarse, dark male-pattern hair distribution. Seventy-five years ago two French physicians described this condition as "the diabetes of bearded women." Name this syndrome_____. (Answer in Appendix)

Pregnancy questions

Q. My wife is five months' pregnant and so moody that sometimes she's borderline irrational.

A. So, what's your question?

Q. Is there anything I should avoid while recovering from childbirth?

A. Yes, pregnancy.

Q. When is the best time to get an epidural?

A. Right after you find out you're pregnant.

Q. I'm two months pregnant now. When will my baby move?

A. The day after college graduation.

Ode to a Mammogram

For years and years they told me. "Be careful of your breasts.
Don't ever squeeze or bruise them, and give them monthly
tests."

So I heeded all their warnings and protected them by law.
Guarded them very carefully and always wore a bra.

After 40 years of careful care the doctor found a lump.
He ordered up a mammogram to look inside that clump.

"Stand up very close," she said, as she got my breast in line.
"And tell me where it hurts," she said, "Ah, yes! There! That's
just fine."

She stepped upon a pedal. I could not believe my eyes!
A plastic plate was pressing down, my boob was in a vise!

My skin was stretched and stretched from way up by my
chin
My poor breast was being squashed to Swedish pancake
thin!

Excruciating pain I felt within its vise-like grip.
A prisoner in this vicious thing my poor defenseless tit.

"Take a deep breath," she said to me. Who does she think
she's kidding?
My chest is smashed in her machine, I can't breathe and
weary I am getting.

"There, that was good." I heard her say as the room was
swirling and swaying.
"Now, let's get the other one." "Lord, have mercy," I was
praying.

It squeezed me from the up and down, it squeezed me from both sides.
I'll bet she's never had this done to her tender little hide!

If I had no problem when I came in I surely have one now.
If there had been a cyst in there, it would have popped by now.

This machine was made by a man, of this I have no doubt!
I'd like to get his balls in there and listen to him shout!!!!!
—Anonymous

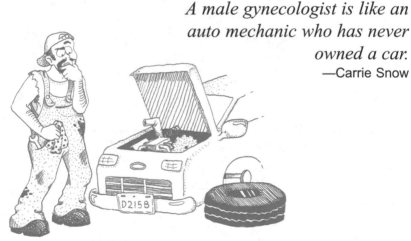

A male gynecologist is like an auto mechanic who has never owned a car.
—Carrie Snow

© Ashley Long

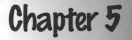

Chapter 5

Snakes, Snails & Puppy Dog Tails

> *Think of sperm swimming upstream. For all but*
> *one of them, it's going to be a very bad day.*
> —Howard Anderson

Sperm tales. A thousand sperm cells are produced every second in the testes. It takes approximately two months to develop a fully mature sperm. After ejaculation, somewhere between 100,000 and 300,000 sperm—give or take a few thousand depending on the season, the scrotal temperature, the length of time between sexual encounters of the closest kind, and a few other variables—make a beeline for the egg, swimming at the lightning speed of 4.2 inches per hour (the equivalent of a swimmer covering 12 yards a second) and reach the site of fertilization within 50 minutes. Sperm live for approximately 2.5 days in the female reproductive tract after ejaculation. The average speed of ejaculation, if you're interested, is 28 miles per hour. If this ejaculation occurs within a closed space, such as a vagina, the force of the ejaculation propels the sperm toward the grand prize, the egg. If, however, ejaculation occurs in an open space sans partner, the ejaculate can be propelled anywhere from 4 to 6 feet in any direction.

The early sperm does not get the worm, so to speak. Contrary to popular belief, the first sperm to arrive at the scene does not get the prize. The first wave of sperm is similar to the infantry on the battlefield. They have been assigned the important function of clearing the way for the "the chosen one." The chosen one penetrates the "zone" that surrounds the egg and drills through the outer membrane in order to fertilize the egg..

How big? Relative to its body weight, the Japanese Dolphin has the largest testicles of all creatures, big and small. The testicles of the blue whale are about 2 ½ feet long and weigh about 110 pounds each. Oh my. The most interesting fact, however, is that the individual sperm of even the largest whale is about the same size as that of a human. In fact, the sperm of a humpback whale is 52 microns in length, the sperm of a sperm whale is 42 microns in length, your basic common porpoise has a 72- micron sperm, and the human sperm is 55 microns in length. So, the testicles might be gargantuan in these larger than life cetaceans, but the sperm is basically the same size. Let's move down a notch to the world of the small, hairy creatures that roam the fields and the plains. The sperm of a prairie vole is the same size as a human sperm. In other words, as a general rule, a sperm is a sperm is a sperm—whether it is an elephant sperm or an emu sperm, with the exception of the humongous fruit fly sperm.

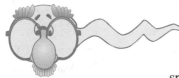

The humongous fruit fly sperm. The October 25, 1994 issue of *The Proceedings of the National Academy of Sciences* has published a report on a special type of fruit fly that produces a single humongous sperm that is several times longer than its body. French researchers at the National Center for Scientific Research stated that if a man could do the same thing his sperm would be 33 feet long. Whoa. Tell me that's a typo. The scientists stated that the size of this fruit fly sperm "almost guaranteed" fertilization. Well, that's a no brainer.

Does size really matter? How can you tell a Y chromosome-bearing sperm (carrying the male DNA in the human) from the X chromosome-bearing sperm (carrying the female DNA) in the human? One way is to see who swims the fastest, and, the Y-sperm is clearly the winner. The traditional theory is that males do *everything* faster to begin with, and that includes swimming. The traditional theory is true; however, there is more to the story. Take a look at the structure of the Y chromosome and the structure of an X chromosome. Obviously there's more to the X…an additional "leg" so to speak. The Y is missing a lower leg. Well, anyone or anything missing a leg is going to weigh less, so the Y chromosome is about 23 to 25 percent smaller than the X chromosome. (This is when all of our weight problems begin, ladies.) We're heavier and we're much slower as a group of swimmers, so the faster you swim, the greater the chance you'll come home with the gold medal, or egg in this case. Male sperm arrive at the scene sooner, which increases the possibility of fertilizing the egg and thus, conceiving a male.

So, let's now say that you have had 12 boys and you want to try *one more time* for the old gipper to have a little girl. Can the weight of the sperm be used to give you a slight advantage? Yes. Researchers can separate sperm according to the size and amount of DNA. They can use the "glow in the dark" technique. By attaching a fluorescent dye, X-carrying sperm glows brighter under the microscope due to the increased amount of DNA. The "duller" male sperm can be separated from the female sperm by using this technique as well. Using this sorting technique, researchers can obtain an 85:15 ratio of the type of sperm desired. Obviously not 100 percent foolproof for the sperm of your choice but close enough so that the odds are in your favor.

If you were work out in human distances how far a sperm has to travel from the vagina through the Fallopian tubes to meet the egg it would represent a marathon swim of over 26 miles.

Historical Highlights

Of course, we have all heard the story of Antonie van Leeuwenhoek, the seventeenth century microscopist, better known today as the Father of Microbiology. His discovery of the single lens microscope over three hundred years ago opened up a whole new world in the realm of science. He observed the world of pond water, tissue from bee stings, and even the plaque between his teeth. But perhaps one of his most incredible discoveries was that of the swirling, whirling, wig-waggling world of semen. A medical student, John Ham, brought him a specimen of "spontaneously discharged semen of a man who had lain with an unclean woman and was suffering from gonorrhea." Ham and Leeuwenhoek both observed "small animals with tails" under the microscope and Leeuwenhoek described these as *animalcula in semine masculine*, ("animalcules" in male human semen.) After observing the specimen from John Ham, Leeuwenhoek decided to obtain semen from a more personal source, but he was quick to explain that the semen was acquired, "not by sinfully defiling himself but as a natural consequence of conjugal coitus." He observed a multitude of "animalcules," that he described as less than a millionth the size of a coarse grain of sand and with thin, undulating transparent tails, which we know today as sperm.

Easier ways to determine the sex of your offspring. Other creatures, big and small, determine the sex of their offspring in many unique ways. For example, the green spoon worm is "sexless" at birth. The sex of the baby spoon larva is determined by whom the larvae comes in contact with during the first few days of life. For example, if the larvae just so happen to encounter a female first, a male green spoon worm will emerge. If, however, the larvae doesn't meet a female, it settles for being female itself. And, that's it. Story ended. No X's, no Y's, no spinning the sperm to determine the weight and sex of the offspring.

Alligators are just as unique in that the ambient temperature of sand plays a major role as to whether the baby alligator will be swaddled in pink or in blue. If the alligator eggs are buried in cool sand the eggs will be "Allison's" and if the eggs are buried in warm sand, little "Al's" will be hatched. It just so happens to be the opposite temperature where most turtles are concerned—cool sand, Tommy Turtle, warm sand, Tanya Turtle. Exceptions abound in the animal, reptile, insect world, but the above are just a few examples of social and environmental clues that determine gender identity.

Can dietary adjustments increase sperm counts? Men with low sperm counts can pump 'em up by as much as 74 percent in 26 weeks by taking a combination of 5 mg of zinc and 66 mg of folic acid. The study, hot off the seminiferous tubules, from the Netherlands, was published in the April 2001 issue of *Fertility and Sterility*, the journal of the American Society for Reproductive Medicine. Folic acid alone or zinc alone did not work. It had to be the combination of the two. The researchers speculated that the zinc was necessary to promote the absorption of folic acid. The study did not test whether this combination led to an increase in pregnancy rates.

Coca Cola as a spermicide. A study from Harvard Medical School may provide a simple, cheap method of contraception. Harvard researchers decided to test the effect of soft drinks on the viability of sperm. They compared the effects of Diet Coke, Caffeine Free New Coke, New Coke, and Coke Classic. Each type of Coke killed the little guys; however, there were significant differences in the effectiveness as well as the amount of time needed to annihilate the cohort of sperm. New Coke proved to be the least effective of the five and Coke Classic was the winner by a landslide. It killed sperm five times faster than New Coke. Although the Coca Cola corporate offices refuse to endorse their product as a spermicidal agent, perhaps this explains the use of Coca Cola as a popular post-coital douche in years past.

Pumpin' the pedals may do more harm than good—depending on the body part. Don't overdo the stationary bike routine or *any* bike routine for that matter. An Austrian study found that men who are dedicated mountain bikers have quite a few problems with their private parts due to the pressure and trauma to the testicles. The good news is—the reproductive apparatus still works. The bad news is—sperm counts are lower and sperm is less mobile. This all boils down to problems with fertility in this group. How long do you have to ride that bike to have the problems? The guys who rode for more than two hours a day, six days a week were the ones most likely to have sperm count problems. They also probably had love life problems considering how much time they spent pumpin' those pedals in lieu of paying attention to their fraulein. (Ferdinand Frauscher, M.D., Uroradiologist, University Hospital of Innsbruck, Austria, presented at the 2002 Radiological Society of North America, 2002)

But in another study.... In a recent Italian study, men who rode a stationery bicycle for one hour, three times a week for eight weeks reported better erections and more satisfying sex than sedentary men. Exercise increases the ability of the blood vessels to vasodilate, which increases blood flow to the penis. One hour a day seems to be quite beneficial; however, when the exercise was increased to two hours a day, fertility suffered. (Lancisi Heart Institute, Ancona, Italy)

Sperm counts and plastic diapers. Hot scrotal temperatures have been blamed for problems with spermatogenesis for many decades. It is a well-known fact that summertime is a time "when sperm-livin' ain't easy." Let's throw in plastic-lined diapers as yet another possible cause of reduced sperm counts and possibly as an increased risk for testicular cancer.

A team of German researchers hypothesize that plastic diapers may pose long-term problems because of the heat factor. Plastic diapers were designed to be leak proof, and they certainly are. However, this also means reduced ventilation and more infrequent changes. The temperature inside the plastic diaper can increase by as much as two to four degrees Fahrenheit during a febrile episode. Why would this contribute to decreased sperm counts and increased testicular cancer rates, you ask? Well, sperm production is optimal when the scrotal temperature is two to four degrees Fahrenheit *less* than body temperature. This is the reason that the testicles have chosen to take up residence *outside* the confines of the abdomen. Testes that remain inside the body (undescended testicles, cryptorchism) have also been shown to increase the risk of infertility problems later in life and to increase the risk of testicular cancer. (*Archives of Disease in Childhood,* October 2000)

Does a sperm have olfaction capabilities? Researchers at Duke University have found the exact same molecules on sperm as those found in the nose used for smelling the sweet scent of perfume. What the heck does that mean? I have absolutely no idea, but continue reading.

Cologne and sperm tail abnormalities. Researchers have found a link between sperm damage and men's cologne, aftershave lotions and potions, and hair sprays. The specific chemical responsible for the damage is monoethyl phthalate (MEP)(the "ph" in this word is silent, so it's pronounced "thalate"). Abnormal sperm have a tail that is much too long for it's own good. The exact mechanism is unknown but further research is headed your way. Should you stop slapping that manly smelling cologne on those cheeks? If fertility is an issue at this point in your life, you may want to impress your date with a little sperm friendly Irish Spring soap instead of an unhealthy handful of Calvin Klein cologne. (*The Scientist*, January 27, 2003)

The mutant sperm theory of schizophrenia. Women have long been blamed for the development of schizophrenia in their offspring. In fact, the preferred method of treatment in the early to mid twentieth century was to remove the child from the mother's presumed "evil" influence and commit the offspring to an insane asylum.

Now a new theory has emerged, and we can finally put some of the onus on the father. This study, funded by the National Institutes of Health, is the first to link paternal age to a psychiatric illness. The research suggests that fathers between the ages of 45 and 49 are twice as likely to have children who develop schizophrenia. Aging sperm accumulates small mutations that are passed on to their children. The older the father, the greater the risk. Men over 50 were three times more likely to have schizophrenic children than men younger than 25. Overall, about one in four cases of schizophrenia was associated with older fathers.

Schizophrenia, which results from a complex and little understood interplay between genetics and environment, is believed by some scientists to involve several gene mutations. The subtle mutations that occur in aging sperm cells may help explain why the incidence of schizophrenia has remained the same over time and across diverse populations even though people who suffer from the illness are less likely to marry or to have children.

These findings demonstrate that men have a biological clock too. In other words, geriatric fatherhood may not be all that it's cracked up to be, nor is it risk-free for the next generation. (*Archives of General Psychiatry*, April 2000)

If you want a boy, expose your husband to chemical pollutants such as PCBs. Men who are exposed to environmental pollutants are more likely to father boys than girls. Researchers studied 101 families who ate fish from the Great Lakes, which are polluted with a potpourri of chemicals, the most notable being the "hormone disruptors" known as PCBs (polychlorinated biphenyls). The families studied had 208 children, 57 percent of whom were boys. Usually only 51 percent of the babies born are boys.

If you want a boy have sex more often. A Baylor University study reported that ardent couples are more likely to have a male child first. The study found that sperm ejaculated after frequent coitus, such as during a first year of marriage or after men return from war, had more Y-bearing sperm than X-bearing sperm.

Doin' it in December. The Population Studies Center at the University of Michigan compared monthly birth rates in the U.S. from 1940 to1990 to weather charts from the same period. They found that ambient temperatures had an inverse relationship to birth rates. In other words, higher temperatures in July and August resulted in lower birth rates in the following spring. The researchers found that more babies were born in September than any other month, making December the most popular month to conceive. November conceptions came in a close second.

Is there a rational explanation for the findings aside from the obvious? How about that it is just too bloomin' hot in July and August in most parts of the country and therefore any activity that increases the heat and sweat factor may not be as pleasurable, including sexual activity. In contrast, November and December are more amenable to close encounters of the sexual kind when the weather is conducive to snuggling and cuddling.

Another explanation may also explain the findings. As we are all aware, the testicles are located outside the abdomen in the scrotal sac. Remember—location, location, location. Since the testicles are located outside the warm, cozy internal environment of the lower abdomen, they are cooler than the

> **Fact:**
> *The nation's oldest sperm bank is in Roseville, Minnesota.*

rest of the body's organs. The internal temperature of the body is maintained at a fairly constant 98.4° F. Scrotal temperatures are 3° F less, running around 95° F. (When is the last time *you* took a scrotal temperature?) Cooler temperatures keep those sperm-producing cells pumping.

Sperm counts are significantly lower when ambient (environmental) temperatures rise. Conditions where this might happen include the hot summer months, relaxing in the warmth of a hot tub or sauna (hot tubs and saunas may be aphrodisiacs, but they are not fertility enhancers—users beware), and (some have claimed), wearing tight fitting jeans or briefs. All of these conditions increase scrotal temperatures and decrease sperm counts. So, the moral of the story is to coooool down those testicles if you want to increase the chance of conceiving that little bambino.

The number and motility of sperm cells is decreased for up to six weeks after a one-hour session in the hot tub. A 102.4° F temperature for one hour can cause immediate damage to the sperm. Most health clubs keep their hot tubs at 104° F. Fertility is at its lowest four weeks after the hot tub session, when sperm that were immature while sitting in the hot tub finally matured. Is this a permanent problem? No. The average life span of a sperm is 75 days, so all damaged sperm will be replaced within that time—provided of course, that the testicles have stayed out of a hot tub during that time.

Losing virginity in the month of June. Research psychologists from the University of Oklahoma tallied up the answers on 4,306 questionnaires filled out by high school youths. Their findings: Most teenagers (all sexes, all sizes, all races and all colors) lost their virginity in the summer months. June seemed to be the most popular month of all. Possible explanation? The Raging Summer Hormone Theory? The Summer Vacation Theory? School is just out, jobs are scarce, mom and dad are working, hanging out is in, and opportunities abound in the back seat of every Toyota Corolla and recreation room couch.

Removing brassieres can be hazardous to your health. Hey guys, if you're going to be doing it in the back seat of your Toyota Corolla you might as well learn how to remove the lady's lingerie without harming yourselves. Researchers from London's St. George's Hospital in London recommend that men take lingerie-removing lessons before embarking on this pastime. Why in the world would that be necessary? Surveys have shown that 40 percent of men in their 30s and 40s are equally uncoordinated when floundering with clasps and hooks and risk injury when making feeble attempts to undo them. Case in point: A 27-year-old man, after an evening of ribaldry, was having an intimate moment with his female companion. As he was attempting to unclasp her brassiere, he twisted his left middle finger in the bra strap and sustained a fractured middle finger with torn ligaments. Instead of getting to "first base" he had to be admitted to the hospital to repair the damage to his fumbling finger.

The Big T—testosterone toxicity. The definition of masculinity clearly lies in the lap of the omnipotent, all-powerful hormone testosterone. For hundreds of years scientists (male) were convinced that the male body contained a kind of magical masculine hormone. Throughout the ages scientists (male) have attempted to "bottle" this substance by grinding up thousands of pounds of bull testicles, analyzing millions of gallons of policemen's urine, grafting monkey testes onto aging men, and injecting themselves with pureed dog testicles. Ground-up goat testicles were used to treat every complaint known to man (and woman)—from bunions to brain tumors to epilepsy and earaches.

The use of anabolic steroids (testosterone and its derivatives) to enhance physical prowess has been declared illegal by all national and international athletic committees. Of course that doesn't mean that the athletes listen to those rules—after all, it's just a rule. In addition to the condemnation on the basis of fair play (some take steroids, some don't, therefore unfair), the known adverse effects as well as the unknown long-term effects are cited as reasons to ban the use of anabolic steroids.

The number of athletes using anabolic steroids is difficult to accurately assess since it is considered illegal. Kids as young as 10 are using steroids, women report using steroids to enhance their athletic performance, and all levels of athletic competition have reported use—professional, amateur, collegiate, high school and yes, even junior high school.

> *Sex without love is an empty experience, but as empty experiences go, it's one of the best.*
> —Woody Allen

The use among body builders and weight lifters is estimated to be as high as 80 percent. Professional football players are major users (as reported by the athletes); however, coaches and owners estimate that only 6 percent are users. It appears to be a slight underestimation by all accounts. The estimated use by high school male students is 11 percent. Eighty-four percent of the users participate in competitive or noncompetitive sports.

Athletes tend to take doses that are 10, 100 or even 1,000 times larger than the doses prescribed for medicinal purposes. They also cycle the drugs before competition, a technique known as "stacking"—alternately tapering the dosage upward and downward before a competitive event.

Acute effects of testosterone use include euphoria and an increased sense of well-being. As the drug is tapered downward, users report a lack of energy, increased irritability, and dysphoria. The users are also prone to outbursts of violent behavior. As use continues, the toxic effects may be observed in various organ systems including the heart and liver.

A case of anabolic steroid use and athletic prowess. Will the will to excel ever end? When will the doping violations for major sports events cease to exist? Well, it appears as if doping with anabolic steroids is not just limited to weight lifting, wrestling, bicycling, professional football, professional baseball, and professional basketball. It has now entered the cutthroat world of table tennis. Yes, dear readers, the scandal continues to involve athletes in every venue. Table tennis player Barney Reed Jr. of New York has been suspended for two years following a doping violation. Reed tested positive for anabolic steroids at the 2001 North American Championships in Ft. Lauderdale and his suspension is retroactive through July 6, 2001. This, of course, means that his winning results since that time have all been erased from the record books. And, from what I understand, Barney was a mean doubles player in the world of table tennis. Must have been the massive biceps and unfettered aggression.

Monkey T (testosterone), monkey do. Perhaps the most studied of all male testosterone-induced behavior is the male monkey. Levels of testosterone have been measured in all sorts of situations. If a male monkey sees an attractive and available female, the Big Monkey T level shoots up. If another male monkey, of a higher social status, covets the same female monkey, both males have a surge in testosterone as they ready for the battle over the favors of the female monkey. After the males fight, testosterone remains high or may climb another 20 percent in the winner, while the testosterone plummets by as much as 90 percent in the loser.

It appears that testosterone levels can stay elevated in the winner; hence, they retain bragging rights for at least 24 hours. The loser will tippy-toe quietly to the corner and lick his wounds for a longer period of time, *unless* a sexually receptive female just happens to enter the picture and show an interest in the loser. As Dr. Kim Wallen (Emory University, Yerkes Regional Primate Research Center) so aptly puts it: "So now you know what accounts for the popularity of strip bars: they're where male losers go to get their T back up." The levels of testosterone in monkeys have shown that watching anything with a sexual content can boost the T levels in winners and losers. Wind up a monkey porno video and simian testosterone levels soar up to 400 percent higher than prior to "Let's Play Hide the Banana." Boot up to the porno Internet sites and count the 150 million hits these sites receive per day. These sites are a natural for triggering a rise the big T levels without having to swagger into the local strip joint or Hooter's for a burger.

The big T and T-bones. Men who don't get enough protein in their diets may have low testosterone levels and a diminished sex drive. AAAARRRGH!!! One hand beating the chest while the other hand grips the oversized turkey leg, grease dripping down the chin, comes to mind here. Researchers at the University of Massachusetts report that low levels of testosterone can also lead to a reduction in muscle mass, weakened bones, and anemia. No wonder real men don't eat quiche. It doesn't do a dang thing for them. Men need to eat *meat, meat* and more meat, at least to be real men. Does that mean that Vinny, the vegetarian, is not a *real man?* Vinnie! Eat meat! "Yo ma', I dohna wanna eat no meat." Ok, Vinnie, eat other sources of protein such as dairy products and eggs (depending on your type of vegetarianism), beans, soy—yeah, Vinnie, how about a little tofu?—peanut butter, and whole grains. (*J of Clin Endocrinology*, June 2000)

Testosterone levels in married men. Compared to single males, testosterone levels are lower in married men. Teleologically this may be Nature's way of keeping a man monogamous and attentive to his children. Give them too much testosterone and they may be looking for love in all the wrong places. So Mother Nature provides an internal safeguard against the tendency to wander by making sure testosterone levels plummet after saying "I do."

Notes on testosterone levels. Serum testosterone levels are one-third higher in the morning than in the afternoon.

A classic case of testosterone excess…the female hyena. The female hyena provides a glimpse at the critical role of sex hormones during fetal development as well as during early postnatal life. In order to study the female spotted hyena one must be able to physically differentiate between the male and the female. "Oh that's a piece of cake," you say, "just look between the legs for the male sex organ and you can distinguish the two." Not so fast, buster. All hyenas, whether male or female, young or old, possess a long, tubular organ strategically placed between the hind legs. Yes, indeed, gender and age make nary a difference. Every hyena is endowed with what appears to be a penis.

The female penis, however, is a rather unique structure. It has the capacity to have an erection and does so during social interactions with other members of the pack, regardless of the sex of that member. During intercourse, the female penis actually becomes a pseudovagina. With unique retractor muscles located on either side of the penis, the female pulls it up into the abdomen forming a hollow orifice for copulation. (An analogy would be the inverted sock routine—reaching down into a sock and pulling it inside-out gives the same effect.)

After serving as the vagina, the penis becomes the birth canal once gestation is complete. Baby hyenas must traverse this narrow tube to enter the cold, cruel world known as the spotted hyena family. The penis must stretch astronomically to accommodate the size of hyena pups. (Try to imagine the human male giving birth through the urethra of the penis. The concept is painful to imagine—laughing like a hyena does not come to mind.) It comes as no surprise that stillbirths are common due to delivery complications.

> *I never married, because there was no need. I have three pets at home that answer the same purpose as a husband. I have a dog that growls every morning, a parrot that swears all afternoon, and a cat that comes home late every night.*
> — Marie Corelli

Besides the obvious, why is the female spotted hyena so unique? No other species even comes close to this bizarre twist of gender identity. The answer appears to be hormonal. Female hyenas have higher levels of testosterone than any other female species.

A brief digression is necessary at this point. The normal process of gender differentiation requires inheriting either the X chromosome for the girl or the Y chromosome for the boy. From conception through the first two months of gestation it is impossible to determine the sex of the developing fetus when examining the external genitalia. The fetus is "unisexual," having undifferentiated internal tissues that have the capacity to develop into male sexual tissues (penis, scrotum, testes, vas deferens) or female sexual tissues (clitoris, labia majora and minora, ovaries, Fallopian tubes). This gender differentiation is dependent upon the X or Y chromosome.

During the seventh week of gestation a portion of the Y chromosome, the SRY (Sex Region on the Y chromosome), instructs the undifferentiated gonads to produce testosterone. This testosterone triggers the differentiation and maturation of the male fetus. Apparently, the lack of testosterone triggers the differentiation and maturation of the female fetus.

In all species, except for the hyena, fetal hormone production in the male (or lack of hormone production in the female) performs the lion's share of the work in directing the sexual development of a specific gender. Inheriting the X or Y chromosome as well predetermines the sex of the hyena cub; however, the big difference is the appearance of the external genitalia, which is a function of the extremely high levels of maternal androstenedione (a type of testosterone). Maternal hyena androstenedione is converted by the placenta into testosterone. This high level of placental testosterone is transferred into the womb where it bathes both the male and female fetuses during gestation.

This extremely high level of prenatal testosterone has profound effects on the female fetal hyena development. The female cub's clitoris develops into penile proportions and it influences the behavior of the cubs. Spotted hyena cubs, both male and female, emerge from the womb as the most aggressive infant mammals on the face of the earth.

Female hyena cubs have been observed to attack their littermates within hours of birth. As soon as the second hyena is born, the first immediately attacks its sibling. Newborn hyenas sport a full set of incisors upon delivery and will bite the unsuspecting next arrival on the neck and shake the ever lovin' bejesus out of it—unless the younger sib has the gumption to counterattack. These young cubs have been known to fight to the death during the process of establishing dominance. In many instances the fighting occurs before either cub has even had the chance to nurse.

If the cubs are of the same sex and death is not the outcome of the initial skirmish, the dominant cub will prevent the weaker cub from nursing. The weaker cub eventually dies of malnutrition and infection. If the cubs are of different sexes, the dominant cub will "allow" the weaker sibling to survive, but the sibling nurses only when the dominant cub has been satiated. This nutritional advantage provides a size advantage that is maintained throughout the life of the hyena.

You many be wondering why mom doesn't interfere with this vicious sibling rivalry. A unique feature of the hyena birthing process provides the answer to this question. The female hyena typically gives birth at the entry of an abandoned aardvark tunnel. The newborn cubs immediately crawl inward to protect themselves from predators. HA! Little do they know that their worst enemy is their own sister Susie or brother Bruce.

This extreme case of fratricide (the act of killing one's sister or brother), may be the result of the need to preserve the species. Researchers have hypothesized that female hyenas have evolved to become extremely aggressive in order to compete for food and provide enough food for their cubs to insure the future generations. The easiest way to become super-aggressive was to masculinize. It appears as if this has become a case of overdoing it a just a bit. Eventually the female hyena became larger and more aggressive than the male. In the hierarchy of every hyena pack every female is dominant over every male, and the pack's dominant member is invariably female.

These unique features of the female hyena provide a fascinating example of the power that sex hormones can exert over physical development and behavior. Prenatal hormones influence all mammals; however, the amount of hormones and the fact that both the female and male hyena fetuses receive this massive blast of testosterone makes this scenario unique.

In other mammals, including humans, only the male is exposed to high levels of testosterone during prenatal life. If the fetus is female, her prenatal sexual and behavioral maturation lacks the influence of testosterone. At birth, the male exhibits the typical male external and internal genitalia and the female exhibits the typical female genitalia.

The bigger and more interesting question involves the influence of testosterone, or lack thereof, on the development of the brain and behavioral manifestations. Is prenatal testosterone exposure responsible for male aggressiveness and is the lack of prenatal testosterone responsible for female nurturing behavior? Does prenatal testosterone exposure cause males to make sexual advances toward females? Does the lack of testosterone cause females to respond sexually to male advances?

Why don't we ask a laboratory rat for its opinion? Lab rats have sex lives that can be completely manipulated by exogenous hormone exposure. If a lab rat is exposed to a big bolus of testosterone (male or female), the rat will act like a male and mount any and every female in the lab. Without the shot of testosterone, both the male and female lab rats will wait passively for the advances of a testosterone-enhanced male or female.

Human brains are much more complex. At least we like to think we are more evolved than lower forms of mammals such as lab rats. Are human females more nurturing than human males simply because of the lack of prenatal testosterone, or do gender-specific environmental clues given from day one shape the nurturing observed in the human female?

Do imbalances in body chemistry result in violence in young men? Copper and zinc may be the keys to suppressing violence in young men according to a study in *Physiology and Behavior*. Imbalances in body chemistry, specifically an elevated copper level and a depressed zinc level, are linked to behavior disorders in some young men. The study, comparing men with a history of assaultive behavior to a control group with no violent history, revealed that the test group's mean copper:zinc ratio was statistically higher than that of the control group. (*Quantum sufficit*, Am Fam Phys 56(8); 1997)

A healthy penis. One of the most important aspects of penile health and erectile function is blood flow. The penis contains 70 to 100 times as much blood when erect than when flaccid. So, if arteries that deliver blood to the penis are blocked with fat plaques (atheromas), the vascular component of an effective erection is compromised. Enter sildenafil, better known as the little blue pill, or Viagra.

If men can run the world, why can't they stop wearing neckties? How intelligent is it to start the day by tying a noose around your neck?
–Linda Ellerbee

Does size really matter? The following are fascinating phallic phacts:

- **Size range**—From 1½ inches to 19 inches (Long Dong Silver and Supreme Court Justice Clarence Thomas—as read in the tabloids).

- **Race and size**—The smallest penis found in Caucasians is 1½ inches compared to the smallest penis among African-Americans which is 2¼ inches. The largest among whites is 6½ inches compared to 6¼ inches for African-Americans. The average size for Caucasians is 4 inches, and for African-Americans it is 4½ inches.

- **Heredity**—The size of a man's penis is entirely a matter of genes and is *not* related to his shoe size, nose size, or neck size; however, it may be related to the size of his index finger.

Penis size and the index finger. Well, the old myth about penis size and shoe size is just that—a myth. Two British urologists measured the stretched penile length of 104 men and attempted to correlate penis size with shoe size. They found *no* significant correlation between the two variables. Another myth bites the dust. So stop looking at his feet and start measuring his index finger length. A group of Greek researchers measured various aspects of the genitalia in 52 healthy men under age 40 and matched those measurements to other characteristics of men including their age, weight, height, body mass index, waist/hip ratio, and index finger length. The only measurements that were significantly related to each other were penile length and index finger length. The longer the index finger, the longer the penis. (*British Journal of Urology* October 2002; *Urology* October 2002)

The Caramoja tribe of Northern Uganda elongate their penises by tying a weight on the end of it. This procedure works so well in some young men that they have to tie a knot in it in order to not trip over it. The rationale of this ritual escapes me at the moment, but I'm sure there is a good reason for it in this particular group of folks living in Uganda. Tying the knot in this particular part of the world takes on a totally new meaning as compared to our neck of the woods.

Odors that increase blood flow to the penis. Out of Viagra and need a little blood flow? Here are some dietary supplements and possible herbal remedies that might get the blood flowing for one last stand—a sniff of lavender, a snort of a Twizzler (licorice), a box of chocolates, the smell of Dunkin' doughnuts, and perhaps Momma's homemade pumpkin pie.

Tissue engineering update—building a new male member. *What?* Yes, Harvard researchers have successfully removed the corpora cavernosa (the spongy tissue from the penis that fills with blood for the erection) from 18 rabbits and have used cells from this spongy tissue to grow replacement tissue. Since the tissue is from the rabbits' own cells, the tissue wasn't rejected by the immune system. But, did the new penis work? Yes. Once the rabbits were placed in the cage with members of the opposite sex they were able to copulate, penetrate, and produce sperm, all within 30 seconds of entering the cage. Researchers stated that the penis worked about as well as a penis from a 60-year-old male as opposed to a 30-year-old male. Stay tuned.

A little foreskin goes a long way. Here's the answer to that question, "What do they do with all of the circumcised foreskin?" Organogenesis, Inc., of Canton, Massachusetts has been using human foreskin cells to produce human skin grafts for patients with venous leg ulcers and diabetic foot ulcers to patients with multi-thickness burns. One foreskin, the size of a postage stamp, snipped from an unsuspecting neonate, can produce as many as

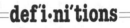

def'i·ni'tions

Priapism is a persistent, abnormal erection of the penis that occurs in the absence of sexual desire. It can be caused by conditions such as sickle cell anemia or spinal cord injury, and is considered an emergency situation when it occurs. Priapus was the mythological god of procreation whose nude statues were well recognized by the size and erectile state of his penis. It has been said that the statues of Priapus were placed in vineyards or cultivated fields as scarecrows.

200,000 grafts. The foreskin cells are separated at birth, so to speak, and multiplied in culture banks. Foreskin actually contains various types of cells, not all of which are useful for skin grafting.

The separation process discards the "immune-stimulating" cells, and saves the fibroblasts and keratinocytes for the culture plate. The fibroblasts help stimulate the growth and regeneration of the dermis of the skin while the keratinocytes provide the protective top layer or epidermis. The fibroblasts are mixed with proteins, such as collagen, from the tendons of the bovine species. It takes approximately six days for the layer of dermis to grow, after which the keratinocytes are tossed into the culture plate. The keratinocytes form the tough outer layer known as the stratum corneum, the layer capable of resisting injury and infection. Twenty days after the initial "snip" in the newborn nursery, the tissue is ready for use. Voilà!

The skin graft is grown in an individual shallow dish approximately three inches wide. This produces a perfectly round ready-to-wear patch of tissue. It takes a grand total of 15 minutes to apply the patch to the area of need (a venous ulcer for example), and bind it with the gauze patch. The graft stimulates the host's tissue to regenerate and heal the vascular ulcer without having to use a patch of skin from another part of the patient's body.

What *do* they do with all of that circumcised foreskin? A personal story. Many years ago, as a junior nursing student, I remember asking the obstetrician, as he was performing a circumcision, "Just what *do* you do with *all* of that circumcised foreskin?" The physician snorted, hrumpfed, ignored my question, and tossed a perfectly good piece of foreskin into the trashcan. Fast-forward 20 years as I was in flight over Missoula, Montana winging my way to Seattle. I happened to be reading a journal with updates in clinical research and the heading stated

> *I knew a man who gave up smoking, drinking, sex, and rich food. He was healthy right up to the time he killed himself.*
> — Johnny Carson

"New Use for Circumcised Foreskin." My jaw dropped as I nudged the guy next to me and said, "You aren't going to believe this but there is now a use for circumcised foreskin!" The man turned to me with a look of panic on his face, most likely thinking that I was some type of a nutcase. He turned his head toward the window, moved his elbow off the armrest, wiggled closer to the opposite side of his seat, and plastered his face to the glass.

So, I decided to call a pediatrician friend of mine and give her the news. We always tried to "one-up" each other with little snippets of news, so I knew I would get her with this one. I picked up the airline phone, swiped my credit card, and made the call. She was with a patient and I insisted that this was more of an emergency than any patient that she might be seeing (hey, it's $16.00 for three minutes on those airplane phones!). She answered the phone with a friendly "What do *you* want? I'm busy." I said, *"You aren't going to believe this one!"* So, I proceeded to tell her about the new use for circumcised foreskin.

Now the guy next to me was getting interested and was saying, "What, what?" I totally ignored him and turned my body toward the aisle.

The pediatrician laughed and said, "Barb, I have known about the use of circumcised foreskin since I was in medical school!" I said, *"No way*! This is brand new information." She said, "Yep, when little kids are born without eyelids they will use discarded circumcised foreskin for grafting on the eyelid." Well, I had to think about this for a few minutes because I had been a pediatric nurse for 20 years and I had *never, ever* seen or heard of a child born without eyelids. But I swallowed her story, hook, line, and sinker. She then proceeded with the end of the story. She said: "The only problem with using the foreskin for eyelids is that when they get older they get a little cock-eyed."

Needless to say, I burst out laughing shortly before I hung up on her. Sixteen bucks spent on airtime for that ridiculous joke with my nerdy seatmate still whining, "What, *what*?"

> **Fact:**
> *The skin of the scrotum and glans penis is the only part of the body (apart from the eyelid) with little or no subcutaneous fat.*

Penile cancer and circumcision. Cancer of the penis occurs almost exclusively in uncircumcised males. Of the more than 60,000 cases of penile cancer that have occurred in the U.S. since 1930, less than 10 have occurred in circumcised men. Obviously circumcision virtually eliminates the chance of developing this malignancy. Before you shriek and schedule your appointment for a circumcision, also know that penile cancer is

Historical Highlights

Prior to 1900 most non-Jewish males were uncircumcised. The shift toward circumcision in this country was most likely the result of the Victorian obsession with masturbation, reinforced by the 1891 article by the British surgeon James Hutchinson, called "Circumcision as preventative of masturbation."

so rare that your chance of developing this malignancy is miniscule.

Note: Contrary to popular belief, there is absolutely no difference in sensitivity between the circumcised and the uncircumcised penis. (Parsons, *Facts and Phalluses)*

Circumcision and sexually transmitted diseases. Uncircumcised men are twice as likely to transmit human papillomavirus (HPV) to their partners than circumcised men. Human papillomavirus causes nearly all cases of cervical cancer. Circumcised or not, men with fewer than six partners in their lifetime are not as likely to have contracted the virus. (Catalan Institute of Oncology, Barcelona Spain)

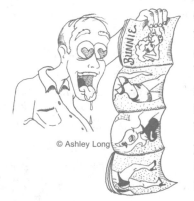
© Ashley Long

Centerfold syndrome. Here's another excuse for not being able to maintain a long-lasting relationship with one's spouse. A psychologist from the VA hospital system has recently described a new syndrome—the Centerfold Syndrome—or the constant bombardment by images of sleek, svelte, perfect female bodies. Men suffering from this syndrome appear to be unable to enter a relationship with the run-of-the-mill, routine, ordinary Plain Janes. In fact, most women, plain or perfect, fail to make the grade with a male suffering from this dreaded syndrome. The researcher concluded that this particular syndrome contributes to high divorce rates, spousal abuse, boredom and dissatisfaction with relationships and marriage. (Brooks, G. Temple Texas VA Medical Center, American Psychological Association presentation, Toronto, Canada, August 1996)

Can the testicles be voluntarily retracted into the lower abdomen? One of the great barroom legends popularized by the James Bond movie, *You Only Live Twice,* was that Sumo wrestlers have the ability to "will" their testicles to ascend into the inguinal canal in their lower abdomen. Moles, hedgehogs, and shrews do it on a daily basis; however, no one is quite sure why. Back to the original story…. In humans, the testes are suspended from the cremasteric muscle, which is controlled by the autonomic (automatic) nervous system. This muscle raises and lowers the testicles as necessary to keep the temperature-sensitive sperm at a constant simmer. Under certain stimuli, such as a cold shower, or more entertainingly a gentle stroking of the inside of the upper thigh, the "cremasteric reflex" takes over and testes are partially retracted into the body. It has been shown that automatic functions such as blood pressure and papillary constriction can be consciously controlled through yoga and the like, and presumably the same could be done with the testicles.

Testicles and endorphins. In the early 1980s, Dr. Candace Pert, a molecular biologist at the National Institutes of Health discovered the group of receptors in the nervous system that interacts with morphine and other opiate-type drugs that we give patients for pain. Once she reported her discovery, her colleagues scratched their heads in consternation and pondered, "Why would we have opiate receptors in our brains? Do we make our own endogenous morphines?" Shortly thereafter, their question was answered. And, the answer was yes; we all make our very own opiates in the central nervous system. The researchers named these opiates "endo" for endogenous, and "orphins" for morphine. Throw the two together and you have the word "endorphins."

My brain is my second favorite organ.
–Woody Allen.

Fast forward to the next decade. Dr. Candace Pert was being interviewed by Bill Moyers for his fabulous book and PBS series "Healing and the Mind." She was discussing the role of endorphins and other neuropeptides and how they were released in response to various emotions. She said, and I quote: "We do know that not all emotions are in your head. The chemicals that mediate emotion and the receptors for those chemicals are found in almost every cell of the body. Why, Bill, you would be surprised to know that there are more endorphins in your testicles than in some parts of your brain!"

Well, duh. Does this surprise anyone in the reading audience?

Orchid. Derived from the Greek *orchis*, meaning "like a testicle." Pliny the Elder, the Roman author and naturalist, pointed out 2,000 years ago that the bulbous double roots of the orchid plant resemble the testicles, thus the use of the prefix "orchi" when referring to the testicle.

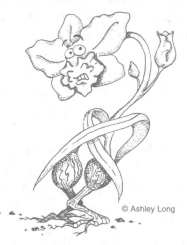
© Ashley Long

- **Orchi**ectomy—the surgical removal of the testicles.

- **Orchi**dometer—yes, there is such an instrument as the ochidometer. And, yes, it measures the size of the testicles. Which of course, begs the question—do testicle sizes vary amongst ethnic groups? And, if the question is asked, the answer must be yes. Here's one that will make you catch your breath: The average weight of the testicle of the Chinese male is 19.01 grams compared to the average weight of the testicle from a male from Denmark, weighing in at 42 grams.

- Crypt**orchi**sm—undescended testicles. When a male embryo is developing, the testicles actually "start" in the area of the upper pole of the kidney. They must make their way down through the abdomen to eventually "live" in the scrotal sac and as they descend they do so via the path of the ureter (the tube from the kidney to the bladder), out the inguinal canal, and into the scrotum. Once they arrive in the scrotal sac, the sac changes its appearance and is said to have the "lived-in" look. If the testicle does *not* descend into the scrotal sac right about the time of birth, the testicles are referred to as "undescended", and it has that "unlived-in" look. This is referred to as cryptorchism.

Peridontal disease and the risk of heart disease. Researchers from the Harvard School of Public Health found that men who had both periodontal disease and 10 or fewer teeth had a 67 percent greater risk for coronary artery disease than men with periodontal disease and 25 or more teeth. Yet another reason to pull out the dental floss.

Sex and men. Why take the time to floss your teeth when you can have more frequent orgasms and protect yourself from heart disease? Men who have the most frequent orgasms have less than half the risk of dying—especially of heart disease. Guys, just 100 orgasms per year can reduce your risk of fatal heart attacks by 36 percent. But who's counting?

Reducing the risk for heart disease by marrying a smarter woman. In the October 2002 issue of the *International Journal of Epidemiology*, a study found that men who married women with college and advanced degrees were much less likely to develop heart disease. A man with a college degree married to a women with an advanced degree had an even greater reduction in heart disease—by as much as 50 percent. A man married to a woman who did not attend college was more likely to smoke, to be overweight and sedentary, and to have high blood pressure and cholesterol levels—all risk factors for heart disease. Why? A few reasons are hypothesized. Educated women are more likely to be knowledgeable about health. They're also more likely to be making the decisions about nutrition and lifestyle. In addition, they're also more likely to have decent paying jobs, easing their husband's financial burden and reducing stress levels. Bottom line: If you want to be healthy for

> *Sex after ninety is like trying to shoot pool with a rope. Even putting my cigar in its holder is a thrill.*
> —George Burns

the rest of your life, always make a smarter woman your wife. Or of course, you can always stay single and just floss your teeth regularly.

Consider the bald man at risk for heart disease. In a recent *Archives of Internal Medicine* article (160:165, 2000), Harvard researchers studied nearly 20,000 physicians and their patterns of hair loss. The men with some frontal baldness at the temples by age 45 were found to have an approximately 10 percent increased risk of developing angina, an MI, or to have had coronary bypass surgery during the 11-year follow-up period. Those who had "vertex-pattern" baldness (loss of a roundish patch of hair on top of the head) had a 25 percent risk of developing coronary artery disease during the 11-year follow-up time. Men with a combination of vertex pattern baldness *and* hypertension were almost 75 percent more likely to develop a serious coronary problem.

The perils of being portly. In a survey of 1,981 men aged 51 to 88, 24 percent reported moderate to severe erectile dysfunction (ED). The men with ED were more likely to be older, have hypertension, and weigh more than their study counterparts. Men with waistlines measuring 42 inches were found to be twice as likely to suffer from ED compared with men whose girth measured 32 inches. Men who were sedentary were also twice as likely to suffer from ED as men who exercised at least 30 minutes per day.

The stamp test. There are many causes of erectile dysfunction (formerly known as impotence) in the male. The causes include vascular problems such as atherosclerosis, neurologic problems including diabetes, pharmacologic agents including antihypertensive drugs, low testosterone levels, and psychological causes. One of the ways to differentiate between psychological causes of erectile dysfunction and all of the other

Live a Little, Laugh a Lot

causes is to perform the "scientifically-based" test known as the stamp test.

The stamp test is based on the fact that all men have erections during sleep. In fact, these occur during rapid eye movement sleep (REM sleep) and most men have five to seven episodes of REM sleep per night, resulting in five to seven erections during the night—*if* everything is in working order. Nocturnal erections can only occur if all of the physiologic parameters are in functioning order—especially adequate blood flow and neurologic function. If the individual can experience erections during sleep then most likely the problem is during wakefulness, and this would be due to a psychological ("I don't think I can do it") problem. So, how can one determine whether or not it's psychological impotence without staying up all night and watching "it"?

Simple. As soon as you finish this section, bolt over to your friendly local post office and purchase six 1-cent stamps. Don't tear the stamps apart—you want them all attached in a nice little row. Prior to bedtime, lick the stamps and wrap them around the base of the penis. Now, everyone go to sleep, and when you awake, yank the covers off and see what has happened to the stamps. If the stamps have pulled apart then obviously everything is in working order—plenty of blood flow and the nerve to do it. So, most likely the problem is right smack dab in the head, and psychological impotence can be diagnosed.

P.S. I told this story in one of my seminars and a woman from the back of the room raised her hand and said, "What if I don't want to spend six cents on him?" Someone else from the other side of the back of the room hollered out—"Use your Christmas Seals!" I guess we all have about six of those left over from a Christmas past, eh?

Male contraceptive—Reversible Inhibition of Sperm Under Guidance (RISUG). Wow! Sounds like it's right outta' Star Wars! The new technique injects a polymer into the vas deferens. The drug coats the walls of the vas deferens and the sperm are zapped as they pass through the tube on the way out. The procedure, now only available in India, takes ten minutes and involves no hormones. Unlike a vasectomy, flushing out the drug with the injection of a solvent can reverse RISUG. The only side effect reported thus far is an initial swelling of the scrotum after the procedure. The contraceptive effects of the drug last six to fifteen years. Injections performed ten years ago are still working as we speak. The optimal time to re-inject has not been worked out yet.

Testis. Testis is the Latin word for "witness." In ancient times, the person bearing witness grasped the scrotum, presumably his own, but on occasion someone else's within grasping distance, to validate the testimony. Hence, to "testify."

A British ad for Dr. White's Towels and Tampons reads:
Have you ever wondered how men would carry on if they had periods? If men had periods the cry would go up for the 3-week month, never mind the 5-day week.

The ad goes on to say:

We aren't naïve enough to imagine we could make your period a lot of laughs, exactly. But we're certain we can make it less of a (dare we say it?) bl**dy nuisance."

With severely ill men over 75 years of age who are hospitalized, the absence of one or both hands on their genitals is a grave prognostic sign.
—Clifton Meador, M.D.

Chapter 6

Shampoos, Tattoos & BarBQues
What's new in the world of infectious disease?

> *Support bacteria—they're the only culture some people have.*
> —Anonymous

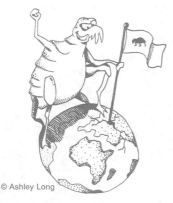

© Ashley Long

Anthrax. Anthrax spores are resistant to sunlight, heat and disinfectant, and can remain active in soil and water for years. Anthrax has killed farm animals (most often sheep, goats, cattle, horses, and pigs) as well as humans for hundreds of years. Most cases of human have been contracted through skin contact, ingestion or inhalation of the organism from infected animals or animal products. Exposure to anthrax from goat hair was known as "woolsorter's disease." Person-to-person transmission of inhalation disease does *not* occur, however direct exposure to fluids from skin lesions may result in a secondary skin infection.

> *When you let the politicians back into the anthrax-contaminated U.S. Senate building, there was enough hot air to kill all the spores.*
> (*Positively Aware,* March/April 2003)

Bioterrorists would most likely aerosolize the bacteria to deliver the organism through the respiratory route. In 2001, anthrax spores were intentionally distributed through the U.S. Postal system in Washington, D.C., causing five deaths. Letters reached the offices of the Senate building and of course our fearless leaders evacuated the building after widespread panic ensued. The case has not yet been solved however the prevailing theory is that this bioterrorism attack came from within our own country. The post office cases followed an initial case reported from the offices of the *Sun,* a supermarket tabloid in Boca Raton, Florida. The U.S. had not had a case of inhaled anthrax for 25 years prior to this case. Perhaps the only humorous anecdote to come from this nightmare was a comment from a physician during a bioterrorism session after the anthrax fiasco:

Historical Highlight

The first anthrax vaccine was given to twenty-four sheep, one goat and six cows. This first vaccine was an attenuated form of the bacteria and was given on May 5, 1881, by a 60-year-old scientist by the name of Louis Pasteur. He gave 3 doses of the attenuated vaccine, each two weeks apart. On the final day, the full-strength, highly virulent strain of the bacterium was given to not only those animals receiving the prior doses, but also a control group consisting of the same number and species. After two days the animals that had not had the previous two doses of attenuated vaccine were either all dead or dying of anthrax. The animals receiving all three doses of anthrax were healthy and thriving.

Bacteria—the numbers. It has been estimated that 5 million trillion trillion bacteria live on this earth. Their combined weight is roughly equal to that of the top three feet of France. Although bacteria live almost everywhere, 94 percent live on the top 1,200 feet of the earth's surface. The bacteria residing within the intestinal tracts of animals and humans accounts for just a fraction of 1 percent of the total 5 million trillion trillion. Bacteria make up 90 percent of the weight of human feces.

There are more bacteria in a handful of soil or inside your mouth than the total number of people who have *ever* lived on this planet.

Bacterial multiplication tables. Bacterial colonies can double every 10 to 20 minutes. This rate of growth is exponential so that a single colony bred under perfect conditions could reach the size of earth in less than 48 hours. *Salmonella* grow best at 100° F (37.8° C), making the human body the perfect host. *Salmonella's* incubation time is six to forty-eight hours.

Keeping food colder than 40° F (4.4° C) or greater than 140° F (60° C) reduces bacterial growth to practically zero.

Bacteria and coffee mugs. A food safety expert at the University of Arizona rounded up 53 coffee cups

Fecal facts: *There are five times more bacteria residing in your rectum than in the rest of your gastrointestinal tract, which includes your mouth. This explains why the rectal temperature is always higher than the oral temperature— there's a bigger party going on below the belt. In other words, the room temperature always goes up with a bigger crowd in the room. This room just happens to be the rec (tal) room. The rectal temperature is approximately one degree higher than the oral temperature.*

Historical Highlight

A fossilized 3.5 million-year-old bacteria was found in a rock in western Australia and it is believed to be the oldest pathogen discovered to this day.

from office kitchens around the campus. Of the 53 cups, 22 were coated with significant numbers of coliform bacteria (the kind of bacteria that reside happily ever after in your rectum and colon, like E. Coli.) Even if the coffee cup looks as clean as a freshly powdered baby's bottom, it can harbor just as many bugs as a baby's bottom—about a pound or two of these coliform bacteria.

© Ashley Long

Bacteria and toilet seats. "If you have a choice between licking the top of a toilet seat and a cutting board, choose the toilet seat!" says Dr. Charles Gerba, a microbiologist at the University of Arizona in Tucson. The kitchen cutting board has 200 times more fecal bacteria (mostly from raw meat) than a toilet seat. Dr. Gerba has swabbed, cultured and tested everything from toilet seats to teakettles to cutting boards and coffee cups. He has found that the cleanest part of all bathrooms is the top of the toilet seat—cleaner than the sink and certainly cleaner than the floor. The underneath surface of the toilet seat would qualify as a toxic waste dump—especially in houses where the seat is flipped up prior to relieving oneself. However the top, where you flop, could be used as a TV tray it's so squeaky clean. When testing the various surfaces in 15 average households, Dr. Gerba found that the toilet seat was always the cleanest site. He has also rated public bathrooms and it comes as no huge surprise that airport and bus station bathrooms rank below pond scum for cleanliness. Hospital bathrooms take the prize for being the cleanest of the public bathrooms. Women's rooms are twice as nasty as men's rooms—that comes as somewhat of a surprise until you factor in mom's dragging children into the ladies rooms. When culturing bathroom stalls, the middle stalls are worse than those on the end. This makes sense as the middle stalls are chosen more frequently than the end stalls. A microbiologist from the University of Connecticut, Dr. Jaber Aslanzadeh, tells it like it is: "A handshake is probably a lot worse than the toilet seat cover." So, the moral of the story is don't hover over the toilet thinking that you will be "cleaner" if you don't sit. All you do is spray the seat for the next unsuspecting rear end. Sit down. Relax and enjoy the moment. Washing your hands is a much greater safeguard against infection than covering the toilet seat. You also might want to reconsider shaking the hand of a man who has just exited the men's room. For obvious reasons.

> *The typical office desk has 21,000 bacteria per square inch versus a toilet seat with 400 bacteria per square inch.*

Bacteria and communion cups. Just when you thought it was safe to take communion... the common cups used in communion ceremonies may be spreading common bacteria. Researchers reporting in the *Annals of Internal Medicine* found bacteria on 12 of 16 communion cups tested. Some of those organisms were harmless but others were the coliform bacteria—notorious for causing diarrheal illness in humans.

There are good bugs and bad bugs in every family of bugs. You can have good apples and bad apples in every family. The same holds true in the world of bacteria. A friendly bacterium with deadly relatives just happens to be *Corynebacterium glutamicum*. *C. glutamicum* is used to manufacture the all-purpose flavor enhancer monosodium glutamate, or MSG. However, the ugly stepsister to *C. glutamicum* is *Corynebacterium diptheriae*, which we all know has wreaked havoc throughout the world for thousands of years causing deadly diphtheria prior to the discovery of the vaccine.

The top three foods containing bacteria. The top three foods containing bacteria in a government survey of bacteria levels on eight popular domestically grown fruits and vegetables typically eaten raw are:

1) green onions (scallions)
2) cantaloupe
3) cilantro

Note: Only 2 to 3 percent of the above foods were contaminated. So, even though these are the top three, bear in mind that the majority of the green onions, cantaloupes, and cilantros of the world do not harbor enough bacteria to have you racing to the toilet bowl. However, it is still prudent to educate the teeming masses (especially the immunocompromised population) about the possibility of contaminated food products. Just remember to wash all fruits and vegetables thoroughly after bringing them home from the roadside stand or the grocery store.

Bacitracin. *In 1943 a culture was taken from a contaminated wound at the site of a compound fracture in a young girl named Margaret Tracy. The culture grew an aerobic, gram-positive, spore-forming bacteria known as* Bacillus subtilis. *Bacitracin is an antibiotic produced by the Tracy 1 strain of* Bacillus subtilis.

Bacteria, dishrags and sponges. Researchers at the University of Arizona cultured 325 cellulose sponges and 75 cotton dishrags taken from households. At the start of the study, the researchers found a million times as many bacteria in the fluid wrung from dishcloths as on toilet seats. So, once again, if someone gave you the choice of wiping your face with the kitchen dishrag or smooching the top of the toilet seat, the toilet seat wins the prize, hands down. Twenty percent of the sponges and cloths cultured *Staphylococcus aureus* and 14 percent cultured *Salmonella. Staphylococcus aureus* causes 1.5 million cases of food poisoning each year and is responsible for approximately 1,200 deaths. *Salmonella* has been linked to over 3,800 deaths per year. Moral of the story? Use bleach to clean your dishrags at least once a week and wipe the surfaces of the kitchen sink and counter daily with a bleach solution. Add one cup of bleach to a sink full of water, throw the dishcloth in and let it soak for 10 minutes before letting it drain. And don't wipe your face with the dirty dishrag.

> *Physicians overprescribe antibiotics—every time your patient sneezes or coughs at least five other patients are cured.*
> –Steven J. Schweon, *Journal of Nursing Jocularity, 6(3).*

Band-Aids and Earle Dickson's claim to fame. We have Earle Dickson to thank for an everyday household necessity that we all take for granted. Earle, a cotton buyer for Johnson & Johnson, and his wife Josephine, a homemaker, can take a bow for the invention of the Band-Aid.

The Dickson's Band-Aids were literally long "bands" of surgical tape with gauze pads placed every two inches. Textured crinoline was pressed over the gauze and sticky portion of the tape and the bands were rolled up into 18-inch lengths. All you had to do was cut off the length of Band-Aid needed. Since their invention in 1920, over 100 billion Band-Aids have been sold around the world.

Band-Aids with brains. Researchers at the University of Rochester are developing a bandage that will change color if the wound becomes infected with certain bacteria. The bandage will be equipped with a silicon chip programmed to detect the most common bacteria and alert patients as to when they need to see a health care professional for treatment. The bandage is designed for use on any type of wound— cut, scrape, puncture—you name it. And, the makers of the smart bandage are developing software that will enable the patient to scan the bandage at home and thus identify the bug infecting the wound. The software will connect to an online medical database and the type of treatment will pop up on the screen. How cool is that? Of course, this bandage and software are light years away from the shelves at Wal-Mart, but hey, we've come a long way from the days of Earle and Josephine Dickson.

Blood transfusion safety—an update. The blood supply in the U.S. is safer now than *ever*. In fact, blood transfusions today are as safe as, if not safer than many commonly prescribed medications. The tiny risks for viral infection from transfused blood are now estimated as follows:

- 1 in 677,000 units for HIV

- 1 in 103,000 units for HCV (Hepatitis C virus)

- 1 in 63,000 units for HBV (Hepatitis B virus)

- (*JAMA* 2000 July 12; 284:229-35 and 238-240)
  Every day, about 14,000 people worldwide become infected with the AIDS virus known as HIV (Human Immunodeficiency Virus). The vast majority of new infections today are via sexual contact, *not* from contaminated blood transfusions.

"Breakbone fever." This infectious disease is carried by a mosquito. One of the hallmarks of this disease is musculoskeletal pain so severe that it is sometimes referred to as "breakbone" fever. What is the medical name of this disease? _____. Answer in Appendix.

The last major outbreak in the U.S. of "breakbone" fever was in 1985 in southeast Texas after a major order of used tires (approximately 70,000) arrived in Houston from either Nagasaki, Japan or Kobe, Japan. It just so happened that the mosquito *(Aedes egypti)* that carries "breakbone" fever hitched a ride in the used tires of that shipment.

Your next question might just be: Why in the world would Houston, Texas order used tires from Japan when all they would have to do is call their neighbors—as in Arkansas, Oklahoma, or Louisiana?

Actually there is an answer to the question as to why Houston would order used tires from anywhere in the world and not just ask the friendly states to the east and north for a donation. It appears as if Houston, Texas is the "retread" capital of the world and many countries recycle their used tires by sending them to Houston for this purpose.

Botulism. Botulism comes from the Latin term "botulus," or "sausage." The word refers to a toxic condition first observed in Germany in the 1800s after eating sausage. The poisonous substance was called "botuline," or "a derivative of sausage." Not until the end of the nineteenth century was a bacterial source identified and named *Bacillus botulinus*. It is now referred to as *Clostridium botulinum*. The bacterium produces a deadly toxin. In fact, a 12-ounce glass of this toxin has the potential to kill every human being (somewhere in the neighborhood of 6 billion) living on the face of the earth.

Fast forward to today's world of medicine—the Botulism toxin has many uses. Known as Botox, physicians use it to reduce the spasticity of muscle groups following a stroke, in children with spastic cerebral palsy and in patients with spasticity as a manifestation of multiple sclerosis. It is also being used to reduce the rigidity of muscle groups in patients with Parkinson's disease. Botox injections into the forehead muscles have reduced wrinkling of the "furrowed brow" with one expected result—a younger appearance, and one unexpected result being a reduction in the occurrence of migraine headaches.

Historical Highlight

The following is an excerpt taken from the December 1850 issue of *Scientific American* about poison sausages:
"German sausages are formed of blood, brains, liver, pork, flour, etc., and, with spice, are forced into an intestine, boiled and smoked. If smoking is not efficiently performed, the sausages ferment, grow soft and slightly pale in the middle; and in this state they cause, in the bodies of those who eat them, a series of remarkable changes, followed by death. The poisonous power of fermenting sausages depends, first, on the atoms of their organic matter being in a state of chemical movement or transposition and, second, that these moving molecules can impart their motion to the elements of the blood and tissues of those who eat them, a state of dissolution analogous to their own. Organic matter becomes innocuous when fermentation eases; boiling, therefore, restores poisonous sausages, or being steeped in alcohol."

Botulism, aluminum foil, and baked potatoes—a deadly combination. Contrary to popular belief, not all food poisoning due to botulism is due to improper home canning.

Potatoes, like all vegetables that are grown underground, can be easily contaminated with *Clostridium botulinum,* the agent that causes botulism poisoning. Washing, scrubbing, and proper cooking can usually kill the spores of *C. botulinum*; however, when potatoes are wrapped in aluminum foil, the foil reflects heat and prevents the potato from getting hot enough to kill all bacterial contaminants. Paradoxically, the heat kills off competing bacteria, making it easier for the *C. botulinum* to grow. Moreover, foil-wrapped potatoes kept at room temperature provide an oxygen-free environment needed for germination of the spores that cause botulism symptoms. Next time a baked potato arrives on your plate in aluminum foil you may want to think twice about consuming it. (*Environmental Nutrition*, January 1999; *The Journal of Infectious Diseases*, July 1998)

Botulism and honey—a "no-no" for infants. Eating honey in both natural and processed forms, can lead to serious disease and even death in infants. Because of the environment in which it's produced, unprocessed honey often contains spores of *Clostridium botulinum,* the bacterium that causes botulism. The same can be true for processed honey. In most humans, the spores cause no problems; immune cells in the GI tracts of older children and adults release binding proteins that neutralize the toxin. The GI tracts of children under one year of age are too immature to produce the proteins needed to neutralize and destroy the toxin. Once the toxin enters the bloodstream after being absorbed through the GI tract, it binds to receptors on skeletal muscle and results in paralysis. Within hours of ingesting the contaminated honey, infants become lethargic, flaccid and can develop respiratory arrest. If the diagnosis is made early, the prognosis for a full recovery is excellent.

**Bubonic plague or the Black Death (*Yersinia pestis).* The plague of the fourteenth century was referred to as 'The Black Death', and was considered the most devastating single epidemic of all time, killing approximately one-third of the population of Europe and Asia. It originated in central Asia and killed 25 *million* people before it reached

Constantinople in 1347. From Constantinople it was spread around the Mediterranean by merchant ships and by crusaders returning from the Middle East. By 1350 it had spread throughout Europe, and at least another 25 million people died. Another major outbreak occurred in 1665 and killed tens of thousands of Londoners. Bubonic plague is rare in the U.S. Since 1944 there have only been 362 documented cases here, primarily in the Western states.

The most recent case of bubonic plague in the U.S. About 10 to 40 cases of bubonic plague occur in the U.S. annually, almost half of which are in Santa Fe County, New Mexico. The bacteria that causes bubonic plague is transmitted by fleas, which attach themselves to wild

---

A Nursery Rhyme

Ring around the rosy,
A pocket full of posies.
Ashes, Ashes,
We all fall down.

An innocent children's rhyme sung while marching around in a circle. However, the rhyme was about the Black Plague that decimated the population of Europe in the mid seventeenth century. Between 1664 and 1665 over 70,000 people died in London alone from the Black Plague also known as the bubonic plague.

The first line, "Ring around the rosy" or "Ring-a-ring of roses," describes the first symptom of the disease: a rosy rash that covered the patient's body. The second line, "A pocket full of posies, " refers to the herbs or flowers people carried in their pockets to protect themselves from evil demons that were believed to contribute to the disease. Physicians would wear a beaked mask containing pleasant smelling flowers and herbs to cover the stench of death. The third line, "Ashes! Ashes!" was originally, "A-tishoo! A tishoo!" and referred to the respiratory symptoms with violent coughing and sneezing. And, the last line, "We all fall down," describes the victim's collapse from the disease, with shock and death to follow.

> *Fifty kilograms of* Yersinia pestis, *the bacteria that causes bubonic plague, aerosolized over a city of 5 million people, would result in 150,000 infections, at least 75,000 of which would require hospitalization, and approximately 36,000 deaths.*

animals. The bacteria are known as *Yersinia pestis.* The high concentration of infections near Santa Fe apparently results from a large population of rodents, including prairie dogs and squirrels, which for years have carried infected fleas. A patient with bubonic plague was admitted to Beth Israel Medical Center in New York City on November 7, 2002. His wife may also have bubonic plague; however, person-to-person transmission is rare and only occurs via direct contact with a draining lesion. The last known case of person-to-person transmission in the U.S. was in 1925. The hospital spokesperson confirmed that the patient had recently traveled to New York from a rural area in Santa Fe known to have rodents and fleas infected with the bubonic plague.

Bubonic plague, dental pulp and DNA. *Yersinia pestis,* the bacterium that causes the ancient scourge known as the bubonic plague, killed 75 percent of the European population over the period of 100 years. The evidence strongly suggests *Yersinia pestis* as the causative pathogen for bubonic plague; however, the actual microbe has never been cultured from the remains of victims of the plague. Scientists have finally succeeded in doing so by probing the dental remains of victims whose disease resembled bubonic plague and died as far back as 408 years ago.

Researchers from the University of the Mediterranean in Marseilles, France, recently gathered skulls from two mass graves—one dug in 1590 and the other one in 1722—in which victims of the plague from two nearby hospitals were buried. They removed unerupted teeth from jawbones and examined the dental pulp for genetic material. The ancient teeth from people who died of nonplague causes had no signs of the *Yersinia pestis* gene, whereas 6 of the 12 teeth from the presumed plague victims did contain DNA from the pathogen. The scientists suggest that examining the dental pulp of teeth for various types of pathogens may help resolve the causes of other epidemics in history.

(*Proceedings of the National Academy of Science,* October 27, 1999)

The first bubonic plagues. The earliest unequivocal epidemic of bubonic plague in the Mediterranean occurred in Libya, Egypt, and Syria in the first century A.D. However, the Great Plague of Athens was described by Thucydides in 430 B.C. The symptoms described during this plague however, could have been interpreted as smallpox, typhus, the bubonic plague, or even the Ebola virus causing a hemorrhagic bleeding disorder. (Kohn, GC. *Encyclopedia of Plague and Pestilence.* Facts on File, Inc. 1995)

Fewer than 10 percent of the counties surveyed by the National Association of Counties said they are prepared to respond to a bioterrorism attack. The group reported that one county in Iowa, which it wouldn't identify, had a three-point plan: 1) call for help, 2) hope someone comes, 3) stack bodies in school gym. Yikes. (USA Today, *January 29, 2002*)

Bubonic plague and germ warfare. The ancient Egyptians were believed to be the first credited with practicing of germ warfare, using diseased corpses to contaminate the food and water supplies of their enemies. The plague was also a popular agent of biological warfare in the fourteenth century. In 1346 the Tartans tossed dead plague victims over fortress walls with obvious intentions of infecting all those within the walled cities.

Bugs for breakfast. Every year, 76 million Americans get sick from something they eat: 300,000 of these people are hospitalized, and 5,000 die. (Centers for Disease Control, November 2002)

Catnip and the roach. Researchers from Iowa State University have found that as attractive as catnip is to cats, it's just as repulsive to roaches. Toss a little catnip into a roach-infested cabinet and they will scatter as if a nuclear bomb had been dropped in their midst. The only problem is, it doesn't decimate the pesky critters, it only scatters them— but hopefully to the apartment next door.

So you think you're sleeping alone? After collecting dust samples from beds in 800 homes, U.S. Government researchers found dust mite droppings in excess of 2 mg per gram of dust, a level known to trigger allergies, in 44 million homes. In half of these homes they were five-fold higher—enough to keep you wheezin' and sneezin' into the next century. So, what to do? Turn that humidifier on, wash those sheets in scalding water, and zip up those duvet covers and pillows in allergy-proof covers. Whew! You're safe again…oops…not so fast. The U.S. government researchers also found another friend in bed with you. Cockroaches and their excrement are present in approximately 6 million household beds. And, cockroaches with their dander (skin cells) and their excrement are also potent allergens. You'll *never* sleep alone, again. (American Lung Association/American Thoracic Society Meeting 2000)

Sex and immunity. Well, if you happen to be sleeping with your spouse, significant other, or insignificant other, you might as well have a little hanky-panky. Researchers at Wilkes University in Wilkes-Barre, Pennsylvania, have discovered that people who have sex once or twice weekly have substantially higher levels of the antibody IgA than do people who hop in the sack less than once a week or never at all. IgA is the secretory antibody found in body secretions. It inhibits viral attachment to mucous membranes and therefore protects one from viral infections. It seems to be a roundabout way to increase immunity. Exercise and humor are two other ways to boost IgA—you make the choice.

Chickenpox. Chickenpox is not called "chicken" pox because it comes from chickens. The term, "chicken" has been used for centuries for connotations that mean "weakness" or pettiness, as in "chicken-hearted" and "chicken-feed" and in "ya' big ol' chicken."

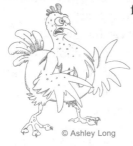
© Ashley Long

Dr. William Heberden (1710-1801), an English physician, used the term to distinguish the typically mild or "weak" clinical course of chickenpox from the more virulent course of smallpox.

Cholera and diarrhea. In patients with cholera, each one thousandth of a quart of diarrhea, of some 20 quarts produced *daily* with this disease, contains 100 million bacteria. If one cholera victim has diarrhea in a body of water, e.g., a river or swimming pool for that matter, the bacteria, *Vibrio cholerae,* will be easily spread to the rest of the community whether they are bathing in the river or swimming in the pool.

Cholera prevention and the use of an old sari. After reading the above vignette you can imagine that 20 quarts of diarrhea a day could be life-threatening if fluids weren't replaced at a similar rate. True, and in third world countries such as Bangladesh, where bathing in rivers is routine, cholera kills thousands each year from severe diarrhea and dehydration. A new study, with lead researcher Rita Colwell, the guru of cholera research and head hauncho

def'i·ni'tions

Pox is actually a variation of the spelling of the plural "pock." The single term is "pockmark." "Pock" most likely originated from the French term *poque* which means "pouch" and its diminutive form *poquet,* or "little pocket." In the Middle Ages any pustular eruption was called "the pox." The smallpox was so called for two reasons—one because the pustular eruptions were small, but most likely because it needed to be differentiated from the "great pox" or syphilis. So, the smallpox was considered to be the lesser of two evils, so to speak.

Historical Highlight

George Washington suffered from recurrent bouts of dysentery (a polite word coined by Hippocrates for the "bloody runs"). George's dysentery was exacerbated by a severe case of hemorrhoids that required him to ride with pillows on his saddle. Since we have been so obsessed with his so-called wooden teeth, we didn't realize the discomfort he experienced at the posterior end of his gastrointestinal tract. By the way, let's put the wooden teeth myth to rest. George's teeth were made from the finest hippopotamus ivory and elephant ivory. (The Samuel D. Harris National Museum of Dentistry)

Dysentery, also known as "campaign fever," was the bane of existence to every military leader throughout the world. More conquering heroes were incapacitated by contaminated food and water causing diarrheal illness than from military force. During the Civil War, the Union Army lost 81,360 soldiers to dysentery and typhoid—only 12,083 fewer than those killed in combat.

Japanese bacteriologist Kiyoski Shigu discovered *Shigella dysenteriae*, one of the major causes of "the bloody runs," in 1898.

of the National Science Foundation in Virginia, has found a simple solution, albeit brilliant. Her 3-year study found that folding an *old* sari into a 4-layered filter can remove more than 99 percent of the cholera-causing bacteria. The older the sari the better. The bacteria cling to the small plankton that feed in the rivers and the plankton are too large to fit through the old, frayed strands of the sari. So the water sans plankton filters through the old sari and the bacteria is "filtered" out with the plankton. This technique cut cholera infections by 50 percent and doesn't cost a penny.

Condom. The condom conundrum would be a better term for this little sac of prevention. The invention of the condom has been attributed to Dr. or Colonel Condom, a seventeenth century English inventor who is said to have produced the first condom from using an inverted cecum (the terminal end of the small intestine) from a sheep. However, long before the Colonel, men were sheathing their "member" in order to fend off the evil "great pox" (syphilis) as well as other poorly understood sexually transmitted infections. One of the most memorable was none other than Dr. Gabriel Fallopius, eponymously famous for naming the female "tubes" after himself, the fallopian tubes. Dr. Fallopius designed a linen cap impregnated with oil to fit over the penis in order to protect him from the great pox in the sixteenth century. Unfortunately the linen cap was not infallible—dear old Dr. Fallopius succumbed to the ravages of syphilis.

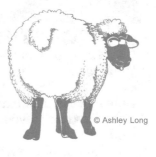

© Ashley Long

Gabriel's bulky oil-impregnated linen cap was unacceptable to many and was changed to fish skin sacs. Dr. or Colonel Condom (by the way, no one is quite sure if he actually was a physician, hence the two designations) has been given credit for changing the material used to cover the penis to the sheep or lamb's cecum. Today these condoms are known as "skin condoms" or "natural feel condoms" and continue to be made from a lamb's cecum. These condoms are thought to produce a more "natural feel" than the traditional latex condom, and are the only form available for those allergic to latex. Unfortunately this type of condom has large pores (up to 1.5 microns in size). This is smaller than a sperm, and smaller than the size of the Hepatitis B virus, but larger than the AIDS virus. So these "Fourex Natural Skins" and "Trojan King-Tite Natural Lambs" may keep the sperm from finding the prize, but they are risky for the prevention of sexually transmitted infections.

Latex condoms and protection from sexually transmitted infections (STIs). The likelihood of becoming infected during a single act of unprotected intercourse with an infected person is estimated as 0.1 percent for HIV, 20 percent for gonorrhea in men and 30 percent for syphilis in men. In women, the infectivity rate during a single act of unprotected intercourse is 50 percent for gonorrhea, 50 percent for human papilloma virus (HPV) and 70 percent for chancroid.

For individuals who do not wear condoms the likelihood of acquiring an STI from an infected partner increases rapidly with the number of coital exposures for infections with high infectivity rates but remains low for infections with low infectivity rates. When condoms are used 100 percent of the time and the infectivity rate is high, the risk for STI

A 1920s condom vending machine bears this message: "Should the presence of this machine be offensive to you, visit our hospitals, health institutes, and asylums. You will be astounded. You may well place the blame upon yourself and others who think as you do."

increases slowly but eventually reaches high levels. For example, the relative risks for chancroid are 0.19 and 0.88 after 10 and 100 coital contacts, respectively.

Hypothetically, if risks are conceptualized with one infected partner and the couple was to begin having twice-weekly, unprotected sex on January 1, 2003, the uninfected partner would acquire syphilis, gonorrhea, and chlamydia in January of that same year and HIV by December of 2003. If condoms were used, syphilis and gonorrhea would be transmitted in about 6 months, chlamydia in 2 years, and HIV in 50 years. (Mann, JR, et al. The role of disease-specific infectivity and number of disease exposures on long-term effectiveness of the latex condom. *Sex Transm Dis* 2002 (June); 2:344-9)

The singing condom. The Japanese have invented a singing condom. The base of the condom contains a microchip and works similar to the way a musical greeting card works. When you open it, it plays the old Beatles song, "Love Me Do."

Cuddly bears and not-so-cuddly bugs. Researchers in New Zealand have found that 90 percent of the soft, cuddly toys in several doctors' waiting rooms were contaminated with nasty bacteria. The pathogens come from the kids who play with them while waiting for their appointments. The toys are stuffed in mouths, dropped onto the floor, sneezed on, coughed on, slobbered on, and so on. The next child picking up Slobber-me Elmo is exposed to an entire plethora of pathogens from the last cadre of kids slobbering on that toy.

The research team tested soft and hard toys found in the doctors' offices for several types of bacteria, including the venerable *E.Coli*. Soft toys were much more likely to be saturated with germs, although most were washed at least every two weeks. *"Every two weeks?"* you shriek. Can you imagine the Godzilla germs lurking in the nooks, crooks, crannies, and crevices after two weeks of runny noses, runny butts, and other runny orifices? Perhaps a more frequent wash would dispel some waiting room fears.

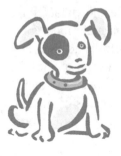

Cuddly puppies and not-so-cuddly diarrhea. Kittens and puppies raised in "sterile" units (puppy farms) have a high incidence of the carrier state for the *Campylobacter* species of bacteria. *Campylobacter* species represent the most common causative agent for bacterial colitis (diarrhea) in this country. When the little precious Peekapoo puppy licks your face, lips, cheeks, and chin, especially after licking their precious little rectal area, they can easily transmit this organism to you and the entire family. Fortunately this group of bugs causes a fairly mild diarrheal illness in those unlucky enough to acquire the infection. So, if a patient presents with mild diarrhea and abdominal cramping shortly after bringing Fifi home, suspect that the patient is sharing a *Campylobacter jejuni* infection with the new Peekapoo. The treatment is ciprofloxacin for five days. The puppy has to be treated too…and, you might want to reconsider those puppy kisses on your face. (Case & Comment, *Patient Care*, February 28, 2001)

Ears versus rears—which is better for temperature taking in babies? Let's put this baby to rest, once and for all. Bottoms win, hands down. In the March 2001 issue of *Archives of Pediatrics and Adolescent Medicine*, a Harvard Medical School study compared a new infrared forehead thermometer with an ear (tympanic membrane) thermometer and the "old-fashioned way," the rectal thermometer. The new-fangled forehead thermometer missed 40 percent of the fevers detected rectally, but was more accurate than the tympanic membrane or ear thermometer. The ear thermometer missed half of the low-grade temperatures and 24.4 percent of the temperatures over 102.2° F (39° C). So, the bottom line (no pun intended): Please advise parents that ac-

> **Fact:** *Dogs lick their genitals an average of four times per day.*

curacy is the best policy, not ease of use. The old-fashioned way beats the new-fangled way and should be used for infants and toddlers who are too young to use the oral thermometer.

Freddie the ferret and the flu. Although a little known fact, ferrets are susceptible to influenza and even serve as an animal model for the laboratory study of this disease. Symptoms are similar to manifestations in humans, and transmission readily occurs between species. Ferrets can also harbor *Salmonella* and *Campylobacter* species in their GI tract. Even though there have been no documented cases of transmission from ferret to human, they should still be considered as a reservoir for these organisms.

Flu shots and heart attacks. No, flu shots don't *cause* heart attacks, however, they might *prevent* secondary heart attacks. A study presented at the 1999 American College of Cardiology meeting suggested that heart patients may significantly reduce their risk of a heart attack if they receive the flu vaccine every year. The study reviewed 233 patients with a history of myocardial infarction that were seen during the 1997-1998 flu season. Receiving a flu shot reduced the risk of a second myocardial infarction by 67 percent.

These data lend support to the theory that a variety of infections can raise the risk of heart disease, most likely because they set off an inflammatory response in the blood vessels that sets the stage for plaque formation. The protective effect for the flu vaccine was only for the current flu season.

Germs in the coin laundry machines. Dr. Charles Gerba, the guru of germ warfare on kitchen cutting boards, kitchen sponges and other spaces like the toilet, has found fecal bacteria in 60 percent of the 100 coin laundry machines that he cultured. Of the 60 percent, 10 percent were found to have *E. coli* that could cause diarrhea. The source was presumably the laundering of dirty underwear.

The good news, the *E. coli* died after the permanent press cycle in the dryer, but the bad news is that some other bacteria were found even after the drying cycle. So, does this mean that you should never use coin laundromats? Of course not, but immunocompromised patients might want to take note and make sure that their clothes go through the permanent press cycle. (Dr. Charles Gerba, Professor of Microbiology, University of Arizona)

Hand washing—how many times must you be reminded? "With the possible exception of immunization," says Ralph Cordell, an epidemiologist at the Centers for Disease Control and Prevention in Atlanta, "hand washing is the most effective disease-preventing measure anyone can practice."

Studies have shown that a single hand can carry around 200 million organisms, including bacteria, viruses, and a few fungi thrown in for good measure. It takes a *full* five minutes of hand washing to cleanse 99 percent of the bacteria from the fingernails, thumbs, palm creases, and backs of the hands. Surgeons have the time to do this, the rest of us do not. So, if you at least want to wash off 95 percent of the bugs lurking in the cracks and crevices of your hands, wash your hands to the tune of "Twinkle, Twinkle, Little Star" (approximately 20 seconds).

A recent study observing emergency room physicians and nurses found that they washed their hands less than a third of the time after touching patients. And when they did take the time to use soap and water, the average wash-and-rinse was a mere 9.5 seconds. The good news—*E.Coli* and other intestinal bugs are the first to go with soap and water. They exit the hands after about 5 seconds of the wash. Plain soap and water also "uncoat" the flu virus, rendering it incapable of infecting cells of the respiratory tract.

Another interesting tidbit—the hand you use the most, the dominant hand, is often under washed. If you're right-handed, your left hand is usually cleaner.

BOTTOM LINE: If you are in a hurry (who isn't?), clean your hands with an alcohol gel fortified with a skin-protecting emollient like glycerin, or wipe your hands with an alcohol-laden towelette. Research has shown that alcohol hand rinses are actually much better at getting rid of bacteria than soap. (Williams, G. The Biology of Hand-Washing. *Discover Magazine.* December 1999; 36-38)

Hand washing and artificial fingernails. Should artificial acrylic fingernails be banned in personnel caring for patients? Two recent studies suggest that the removal of acrylic nails may be prudent when working in high-risk areas such as the operating room and intensive care unit.

One group of Michigan researchers cultured under the artificial nails of 21 health care workers and under the nails of 20 controls. Cultured twice, 68 to 86 percent of the artificial nail users harbored potential pathogens including yeast, gram-negative bacilli, and *Staphylococcus aureus*. Only 28 to 35 percent of the controls were culture-positive. Hand washing with soap reduced the pathogen count only slightly in both groups; however, washing with an alcohol-based gel had a significant impact, especially in the control group. The pathogen rate was reduced to less than 10 percent in the control group, but to only 50 percent in the artificial nail-wearers. (McNeill, SA et al. Effect of hand cleansing with antimicrobial soap or alcohol-based gel on microbial colonization of artificial fingernails worn by health care workers. *Clin Infect Dis* 2001 Feb 1;32:367-372)

In a second study, surgeons were baffled when three patients in a 6-week period developed post-laminectomy *Candida* osteomyelitis. Gel electrophoresis pinpointed *one source* for the outbreak and the infection control sleuths commenced their search. An operating room technician was the "typhoid Mary," so to speak. Among all of the operating room personnel investigated, the only surveillance culture that grew *Candida Albicans* was from the technician. The operating room technician wore artificial nails contaminated with *C. albicans* and transmitted through her gloves to the bone wax she had kneaded during surgery. Unfortunately she had removed the nails prior to the study so the theory could not be confirmed. Circumstantial evidence would have convicted her, however. (Parry MF et al. *Candida* osteomyelitis and diskitis after spinal surgery. An outbreak that implicates artificial nail use. *Clin Infect Dis* 2001 Feb 1;32:352-357)

A study from a London hospital found that two out of every five nurses harbored disease-causing bacteria on the skin under their rings.

Hand washing and restroom use. When asked directly, 98 percent of women claim they wash their hands after using the restroom. When observed directly, only 74 percent actually do. Tsk...Tsk...

Historical Highlight

In the mid-nineteenth century in Vienna, Austria, a young obstetric physician, Dr. Ignaz Semmelweis, made an interesting observation. He noticed that in wards where an M.D. or resident delivered a baby, 600-800 women died per year of childbed fever. In wards where midwives delivered the baby only 60 mothers died of childbed fever. And, when the mother was lucky enough to deliver at home, without the assistance of medical personnel, the mortality from childbed fever was virtually zero.

The prevailing theory at the time was that childbed fever was caused by "bad air."' Some physicians had the good sense to blame it on a nonspecific agent of unknown origin. That so-called good sense made absolutely no sense, but to continue with the story....

Semmelweis, the ever-observant young doctor, noticed remarkable similarities between the death of the chief of forensic pathology and women who died with puerperal fever. The forensic pathologist had stuck himself with a needle during the autopsy procedure and died of an overwhelming wound infection. Most of the signs and symptoms were identical and Semmelweis began to wonder if something from the autopsy lab was contaminating the women who were delivering the babies. Many physicians were performing autopsies when their patients arrived at the hospital to deliver their babies. The physicians would stop what they were doing in the middle of the autopsy and rush up to the labor and delivery room, not bothering to change their lab coats or to wash their hands for that matter. In fact, as the story goes, the dirtier the lab coat the more prestigious the physician.

Semmelweis had an epiphany. The infection of the uterus was caused by the contaminated hands of the surgeons performing autopsies! He considered childbed fever to be transmissible, *not* contagious. The cadaver's "particles" carried by the surgeons were most likely a variety of agents that were responsible for generalized sepsis.

He ordered all obstetricians and their associates to wash their hands thoroughly in a solution of chlorinated water until they no longer smelled like the cadavers they had been dissecting. The results were dramatic. In the months before the mandated hand washing, the death rate from childbed fever was 18.3 percent. One year after the mandated hand washing began the death rate was 1.2 percent.

P.S. Ironically Dr. Semmelweis died of a wound infection in 1865, at the ripe young age of 47. In other words, he basically died of a variant of childbed fever.

Ten dirty digits. *An interesting resolution passed in 1995 by the American Medical Association's House of Delegates was referred to as "Ten Dirty Digits." The resolution was necessary to remind physicians of their professional obligation to wash their hands with an antiseptic between patients to prevent the spread of infection. This resolution was passed shortly after a study was published stating that only 14 to 59 percent of the physicians in the United States washed their hands between patients.*

Hansen, G. Annauer. Hansen's disease (Leprosy). *Mycobacterium leprae,* identified by the Norwegian bacteriologist G. Annauer Hansen, is an obligate intracellular parasite found exclusively in only two hosts. One of the hosts is the human and the second host is (you'll never guess it in 1 million years) _____. (See Appendix for the answer.)

Head butting and HIV. The November 8, 1997 *Lancet* reported a case study where two men came to blows after a car accident. One had his metal-framed glasses on top of his forehead when he was head-butted by the other man, who just happened to be HIV positive, Hepatitis B positive, and Hepatitis C positive. The force of the head butting left an imprint of the glasses on both men and resulted in significant bleeding. Three days after the fight, the man who was the recipient of the head butting tested negative for HIV, however at 14 days he showed signs of acute retroviral syndrome, and three months later he exhibited signs and symptoms of full-blown HIV infection and Hepatitis B. Another reason to just smile and drive away when confronted during a car accident.

Helicobacter pylori. This corkscrew-shaped bacteria has been observed in the crypts of the stomach since 1913, however, it was always considered to be an "artifact" when described by pathologists. Nary a soul could believe that any bug could survive the acid content of a stomach, hence the "artifact" designation. In 1983, Drs. Barry Marshall and Robin Warren, two Australian pathologists, first proposed that this little corkscrew-shaped bug caused generalized gastritis (inflammation of the stomach lining) as well as gastric and duodenal ulcers. They were ridiculed and guffawed right out of the international meeting in Brussels, Belgium, where they reported their findings. Undaunted, they flew back to Australia to gather more data to prove their theory. As the story goes, Dr. Barry Marshall collected a glass full of the little corkscrew-shaped bugs and drank the whole thing in order to infect himself and prove, once and for all, that *H. pylori* was the culprit. Dr. Marshall was quite ill after undertaking this endeavor, but he was able to prove his point and the rest is history.

Hemophilus influenzae. Ever wondered what a bacterium was doing with a name like Hemophilus influenzae? It appears that the bug was found so often in the lungs of people dying of influenza in the 1918 flu pandemic that the researchers first thought it was the cause of the epidemic and thus gave it that name. Influenzae was so named by fifteenth century Italians because they thought the disease was caused by the "influence" of the stars and planets.

The Herpes "Family." Wondering about all of those Herpes viruses? Here's the Who's Who of Herpes: HSV-1 (Herpes Simplex Virus, type 1), the usual suspect in perioral herpes (cold sores); HSV-2 (Herpes Simplex Virus, type 2), the usual suspect in genital herpes; VZV (varicella

def'i·ni'tions

Herpes is derived from the Greek *herpēs*, that appears in Hippocratic writings as the term for a spreading skin disease or eruption. The root word is the Greek *herpein*, "to creep." The Greek *zōstēr* means "a girdle," hence, herpes zoster that creeps around the torso like a girdle. Simplex comes from the Latin word, *simplex*, "simple or plain."

zoster virus), the culprit causing the primary infection known as chickenpox (also known as varicella) and the secondary infection known as herpes zoster or shingles (Hell's fire); CMV (cytomegalovirus), the offender in gastroenteritis and retinitis (in AIDS patients); EBV (Epstein-Barr Virus), the miscreant in mononucleosis and Burkitt's lymphoma; HHV-6 (Human Herpes Virus, type 6), one of the causes of roseola and a possible suspect in multiple sclerosis; HHV-7 (Human Herpes Virus-7), which has yet to have a specific condition or disease ascribed to it; and, HHV-8 or KSHV (Human Herpes Virus, type 8, also known as Kaposi's Sarcoma Herpes Virus), the herpes virus responsible for cancer of the smooth muscle cells of blood vessels seen primarily in patients with AIDS. So, how about that Herpes Family? Don't you love the term "family"? The word "family" conjures up all sorts of warm, fuzzy, sit-in-front-of-the-fire-on-a-cold-winter's- day thoughts, doesn't it? It's as if they all drive around together in a Dodge Minivan prowling for a human host to infect.

Historical Highlight

An English pathologist, Dr. Tony Epstein, and his lovely assistant, Ms. Yvonne Barr, a Ph.D. student, named the Epstein-Barr virus in 1964. Three years prior to their eponymous discovery, Denis Burkitt, M.D. was doing medical missionary work in the east African country of Uganda. He described a childhood tumor that seemed to occur in clusters in various villages and he hypothesized that an arthropod-borne virus caused the tumor. After a chance meeting with pathologist Tony Epstein in 1961, Dr. Burkitt mailed fresh tumor biopsy specimens from Uganda to Dr. Epstein's laboratory in London.

Epstein and Barr cultured lymphoblast cell lines from Burkitt's tumor cells. In a few cells from the first of those cell lines, which they called EB-1, the electron microscope demonstrated herpes-like particles. Once the virus was shown to be distinct from other human herpes viruses such as HSV-1 (herpes simplex virus-1) and VZV (varicella zoster virus), it was named EBV or the Epstein-Barr virus.
Footnote: The childhood tumor was named after Dr. Denis Burkitt, and is known as Burkitt's lymphoma.

Infectious disease tip of the day. Purchase a new toothbrush after the outbreak of a herpes cold sore and/or a sore throat, strep or otherwise, and you'll be less likely to re-infect yourself.

Herpes genitalia or herpes simplex virus, type 2. Since the 1970s, the number of genital herpes infections has increased by 30 percent. This equates to genital herpes in 45 million Americans. Over the same period it has become five times more common among teenagers and twice as common in individuals in their 20s. Herpes infections *double* the chance of HIV transmission between partners. In addition, herpes genital infections can be deadly to the newborn if transmitted during delivery. As many as 90 percent of the people with genital herpes have absolutely *no idea* that they even have this infection. This of course, means that they are spreading it with wild abandon if they are not using adequate protection.

"Hey Doc, can I catch 'hair-piece' from a toe-let seat?" (Translation: "Doctor, is it possible for me to develop a herpes infection from sitting on a toilet seat?") Well, this question has been asked of nurses and doctors for many years. And, there is no simple yes or no answer. Let me explain. First of all, herpes simplex viruses can live for approximately 45 minutes on a toilet seat. Secondly, in order to acquire a herpes infection the herpes virus must enter either through mucous membranes or through an open cut or wound. So, there are basically three ways to "catch 'hair-piece' from a toe-let seat:

1. Having sex on a toilet seat.
2. Having an open wound on your buttocks that comes in contact with active herpes that has been deposited on the toilet seat.
3. Sitting on the toilet seat with your mucous membranes. (And, if you sit this way on a toilet seat you deserve every drop of herpes you get.)

Herpes zoster (Shingles or "Hell's Fire"). Preliminary studies appear to indicate that vaccinating seniors with the same varicella (chickenpox) virus vaccine approved for use in children would provide a *significant* benefit in preventing herpes zoster or shingles. This live attenuated (weakened) vaccine may stimulate a waning immune system in the older population and give it a well-needed BOOST. This "booster vaccination" jump starts cell-mediated immunity and may confer protection against the reappearance of the varicella zoster virus and, as an extra added benefit, reduce the problem of post herpetic neuralgia, a significant problem in the elderly population. (White, CJ. Varicella-zoster virus vaccine. *Clin Infect Dis* 1997; 24(5):753-63. Landow, K. Acute and chronic herpes zoster. *Postgrad Med* 2000;107(7):107-18)

HSV-2 and psychotic offspring. A recent study analyzed the relationship between maternal infections during pregnancy and the subsequent development of psychotic disorders (eg, schizophrenia and other psychotic disorders). The study tested for HSV-1, HSV-2, cytomegalovirus (CMV), toxoplasma, rubella, parvovirus, and chlamydia. There was a significant difference between the mothers of affected subjects and mothers of control subjects in only one of the infections—HSV-2 (Herpes Virus Type 2). This is considered a preliminary study, but the findings are significant enough to pursue subsequent studies. (Buka, SL et al. Maternal infections and subsequent psychosis among offspring. *Arch Gen Psychiatry 2001;* 58:1032-7)

Sex after sixty. Sexually transmitted diseases (STDs) in the 65-plus age group have increased by more than *300 percent* according to a report by British researchers in *The Medical Post,* October 2001. The researchers attribute this rise in STDs to healthier lifestyles, enabling older adults to maintain their sexual prowess, as well as the Pfizer Riser, Viagra, which as we are all aware, enables males to have erections soon after taking the little blue pill. In addition, high divorce rates have tossed more seniors into the dating circles and with the threat of pregnancy being zero, extracurricular sex has become quite the rage. Woohoo! Our safe sex classes will have to commence with Sunday school and finish with the centenarian swingin' singles clubs.

> *Flies spread disease. Keep yours zipped.*
> —Anonymous

Hepatitis C and Vietnam veterans. Hepatitis C infects 1.6 percent of Americans, however, this number is at least four to five times higher in veterans. Some estimates, depending on the population studied, suggest that 10 to 20 percent of the infected Americans are veterans, the majority of which are Vietnam veterans. And, most of them are probably not aware of their status. A 1998 Veteran's Administration study tested 95,447 veterans and found that 31 percent tested positive, and over half of the positive samples were obtained from Vietnam veterans. Why such a high number in Vietnam veterans?

America's wounded in Vietnam received 365,000 blood transfusions between 1967 and 1969, long before blood was screened for hepatitis C. In addition, drug abuse rates were high in the military in Vietnam as was promiscuity. Many Vietnam soldiers also received tattoos while stationed in Vietnam and investigators have linked this procedure to the transmission of Hepatitis C.

The risk of contracting hepatitis C in a transfusion today is 1 in every 103,000. In 1985 the risk of transfusion transmission was 1 in 200. (Viral infections of the blood supply. Editorial. *N Engl J Med* 1996: 1734-35)

Legionnaire's disease. It was a hot July in Philadelphia in the summer of 1976. The Pennsylvania Department of the American Legion held its annual convention in the Bellevue Stratford Hotel in Philadelphia during the week of July 21-24. Within days of the end of the convention (between July 24 and August 1), reports of conventioneers who had developed pneumonia and had died began to reach the headquarters. The search for a cause began shortly thereafter, and it was soon realized that this "new disease" was actually an old disease, but was not recognized as such. The earliest cases of Legionnaire's have been traced back to 1947, therefore it is a fairly "new" disease as far as infectious diseases are concerned.

Legionnaire's disease is an acute infection of humans, principally manifested by pneumonia, occurring in a distinctive pattern of epidemics and is caused by the bacteria of the genus, *Legionella pneumoniae*. These bacteria thrive in water and prefer temperatures higher than the human temperature. This explains their preference for the hot water side of water systems and the recirculating water in cooling towers or other heat exchange devices. Legionella is capable of living for more than a year inside water pipes in their biofilms and then emerging fully infectious once the tap is turned on. Aerosols created by mechanical disturbances of contaminated water such as showers, sinks, toilets, vegetable spraying systems in grocery stores, hot tubs and swirling Jacuzzi's, and the air conditioning duct systems in hotels and cruise ships provide the "mode of transmission." A disproportionate number of sporadic cases are in people who have recently traveled overnight and stayed in air-conditioned hotel rooms.

One way to prevent the transmission of these bacteria is to maintain a temperature of 60° F on the hot water side of institutional plumbing systems. This will stop outbreaks by lowering the concentration of bacteria in the water supply.

The triad of symptoms for *Legionella* pneumonia. Few bacterial pneumonias show the following triad of findings: relative bradycardia in the presence of a high fever (example: pulse of 80 with a temperature of 103.6° F, or 39.8° C), low serum phosphorus in the absence of any obvious cause, and a rise in liver enzymes. The importance of using this triad to diagnose *Legionella* pneumonia lies in the choice of antibiotics—either erythromycin or doxycycline.

Licking wounds and strep infections. How many times have you licked a cut finger or a cut hand? Just slurped that blood right off of that wound? Ick. Even though saliva is supposed to have antibacterial effects (from its nitric acid content), saliva can also contain bacteria such as streptococci. These nasty bugs have been known to cause bacterial arthritis, bacterial endocarditis (inflammation of the valves of the heart), and pockets of pus (abscesses) in other tissues. So, quit lickin' those cuts. It's too dangerous. Clean them the old fashioned way—rinse the cut with soap and water, soak with hydrogen peroxide, and cover it with a band-aid or other type of sterile adhesive dressing. (*N Engl J Med* 2002; 346: 1336)

Lister, Joseph (1827-1912). In the mid to late 1800s, approximately 80 percent of the surgical patients in Europe were dying of infections within days or weeks of the surgical procedure. During this time, a Scottish surgeon, Joseph Lister, was practicing in England and he was intrigued by some of the ideas of a fellow colleague who lived just across the border in France. A war was raging in France (the Franco-Prussian War of 1870-1871) and the majority of their soldiers were meeting their maker from wound sepsis after surgery rather than from dying from heroic acts on the battlefield itself. The French physician with whom Lister was intrigued just happened to have the last name Pasteur. Pasteur was busy convincing surgeons on the battlefield to boil their instruments before using them, believing that this method would reduce the incidence of death by infection from battle injuries and/or the actual surgical procedure itself. Of course he was right, but his ideas seemed extremely unorthodox at the time. Joseph Lister concurred with Pasteur. He proposed that microbes were the culprits in this postoperative infection referred to as surgical sepsis and he recommended and used a solution of carbolic acid, (also known as phenol) which was known to kill bacteria. In fact, its major use at that time was for the treatment of sewage as well as human waste. Lister cleaned his surgical instruments in phenol, he sprayed the air in the operating room with phenol, and he convinced his fellow colleagues to wash their hands in phenol prior to operating. So simple, yet so effective. The postoperative deaths from surgical sepsis declined dramatically during his tenure as chief surgeon. Lister had introduced the concept of *antiseptic surgery* to the world of the operating room. In his honor a bacterium has been named after him— *Listeria monocytogenes* as has a mouthwash, Listerine. You would think he would get a little more than a mouthwash and a bacterium out of this miraculous discovery.

Listeria monocytogenes is a food-borne illness transmitted most often by unpasteurized milk products. As the immune system enters its golden years, the risk of food-borne infections increases. Foods that are easily handled in our 30s, 40s, and 50s can be deadly in the 70s, 80s, and 90s. Our older population should consider a little more carefully whether the food they're eating could put them at risk for an infection from food-borne bacteria. Immunocompromised patients and patients on immunosuppression drugs (transplant patients and cancer patients) are also at greater risk for acquiring active disease. Pregnant women and their newborns also have an increased risk of *Listeria monocytogenes.* A typical patient would be a 65-year-old dairy farmer with type 2 diabetes and renal insufficiency who occasionally indulged in a glass of unpasteurized cow's milk. *Listeria* is also found in deli foods such as soft cheeses and deli meats.

The following foods deserve some thoughtful consideration: Deli meats and other ready-to-eat meat and poultry products; smoked fish such as lox (smoked salmon); refrigerated pates and deli meats such as bologna; hot dogs; soft cheese such as feta, brie, camembert, blue-veined and Mexican-style varieties. Cooking can kill the culprit, but the above foods are not generally heated at home after possible contamination at the processing plant. Symptoms of *Listeria* can range from flu like symptoms to life-threatening meningitis.

Money and bugs. A study of American coins and currency revealed the presence of bacteria, including *Staphylococcus aureus, E. Coli,* and *Klebsiella,* on 18 percent of the coins and 7 percent of the bills. (NY Public Library Desk Reference, 3rd edition)

Piercing perils. One of every five people who pierces a body part has complications. The most common complications include bacterial infections, bleeding or excessive scarring and tearing of the tissue around the pierced part. The tongue and the navel (belly button) are the most likely areas to become infected. The upper ear runs a close third (see below). Acute, local infections are the usual complication; however, tongue piercing has been associated with brain abscesses as well as a blood-borne infection known as septicemia. Ouch. Piercing the tongue has also been associated with chipped teeth and receding gums and life-long mouth problems including tooth loss. Problems with tongue piercing accelerated after having the jewelry in the tongue for more than two years. Chronic infections acquired from unsterile needles include Hepatitis B, Hepatitis C, and HIV. (*Mayo Clinic Proceedings,* January 2002 and The American Academy of Periodontology, www.perio.org , or 800-FLOSS-EM)

Piercing the upper ear. Just about any body part has been pierced these days, but some body parts are more dangerous to pierce than others. So, the perils of piercing the upper ear have now been well docu-

Live a Little, Laugh a Lot

mented in the infectious disease literature. This area poses a much greater risk of serious infection as compared to the traditional piercing of the lobe of the ear. Piercing the upper ear involves piercing the cartilage, which is more prone to infection than other areas because it receives less blood flow for healing purposes. If the upper ear just has to be pierced and there's no getting around it, make sure that the ear is pierced in the winter months as com-

> *You know the hardest thing about having cerebral palsy and being a woman? It's plucking your eyebrows. That's how I originally got pierced ears.*
> –Geri Jewell

pared to the summer months. The summer perils of perspiration, swimming pools and playing in ponds, rivers, and streams increases the risk considerably.

Lyme disease. The town of Old Lyme, Connecticut is famous for having the first clustering of cases of what is now known as Lyme disease. These cases were first described in 1975/1976 when groups of children with what was thought to be juvenile rheumatoid arthritis were noted in three small communities on the east bank of the Connecticut River. Several adults also complained of fatigue, arthritis, and an unusual rash covering their body. Twenty-five percent of the patients recalled a preceding expanding reddened circular lesion, also known as the "bull's eye" rash. This "clustering" of patients piqued the interest of Yale University rheumatologist Dr. Allen C. Steere. He arrived in Lyme shortly thereafter to investigate this group of patients. He found a grand total of 39 patients with the presumed juvenile rheumatoid arthritis. In a town the size of Old Lyme, Connecticut, *one* case of juvenile rheumatoid arthritis would be excessive. And, since juvenile rheumatoid arthritis is *not* an infectious disease he hypothesized that something else must be causing this clustering of cases.

Lyme disease is now known as the most common tick-borne illness in the United States. The ticks feed on white-footed mice as baby ticks (nymphs) and they move on to deer as they develop into their adult life. It is estimated that 15 to 30 percent of all deer ticks are infected in the northeastern United States. The most cases are reported in Connecticut, Massachusetts, New York, Delaware, New Jersey, Pennsylvania, Wisconsin, and Maryland. It has an annual incidence of 0.5 percent in the endemic areas of the upper Northeast and upper Midwest.

Lyme disease was actually recognized as far back as 1910 in Sweden, however it wasn't called Lyme disease. It was described as an "infection" that occurred after a tick bite, but a specific name was not used. A similar disease was described in Austria in 1913, and in France in 1922. The first cases in the United States were actually in the 1960s in Wisconsin and Massachusetts, however the clustering of cases in the mid-70s in Lyme, Connecticut gave rise to the name of the disease.

Burgdorfer, Willie and *Borrelia burgdorferi*, the organism responsible for Lyme disease. In 1981, Willie Burgdorfer, an international authority on tick-borne disease was called in as a consultant. He examined the contents of the digestive tract of the *Ixodes* tick using a technique called dark-field microscopy and found it to be teeming with a slender corkscrew-shaped microbe known as a spirochete. It was classified as a member of the bacterial genus *Borrelia* and in 1984, in honor of Willie Burgdorfer, it was given the name *Borrelia burgdorferi*. Since that time, more than 80 different strains of *B. burgdorferi* have been identified throughout the world.

Lyme disease has caused unnecessary panic in some northeastern towns promoting the nickname "borreliosis neurosis."

Tick talk. Dr. Henry Feder, Jr., a Connecticut physician, found that deer ticks spreading Lyme disease preferred to bite people who are wearing clothes. In other words, they do their biting under the cover of pant legs, shirtsleeves, and socks. To confirm his findings he *forced* himself to attend a nudist camp for a day or two. He surveyed 300 visitors to the nudist camp as well as the residents and found that the nudists did not receive one tick bite. Those visitors who did not remove their clothes were the only ones who received bites.

Tick-talk. They're miniscule. They have eight-legs.* And, they're blood thirsty. Ticks are arachnids and belong to the same family as spiders and scorpions. The 82 species of ticks native to the U.S. cause at least *nine* different disorders in people and a plethora of diseases in animals.

*A BRIEF DIGRESSION, IF I MAY. You might think that eight legs would not really be a useful number to have hanging off a torso. However, the eight legs of a tick come in awfully handy when scoping out their next meal. Ticks quietly crawl up the side of a blade of grass and hang on with two of the eight legs, leaving the other six free to latch onto an unsuspecting passerby.

It's not really the tick's fault that you acquire the disease from them. Ticks are only passing along pathogens they have acquired during previous feeding frenzies on other infected mammalian hosts, such as deer or rodents. The tick is the perfect vector. It chows down on one host, acquires the infectious particle via the blood meal, turns around and feeds on another host and transmits the pathogen to the next guy. How rude. But hey, that's part of livin' large in the world of ticks. In fact, ticks are perfectly designed vectors. They are tiny (in their nymph stage they are about the size of a straight pinhead), and they live a long hearty life. In fact, some ticks can live for up to15 *years* between blood meals. Humans can barely make it 15 *minutes* before our thoughts turn to the next happy meal.

The black-legged tick (*Ixodes scapularis,* or *Ixodes dammini)* formerly known as Prince, just kidding…formerly known as the deer tick, and the Western black-legged tick (*Ixodes pacificus)* most often carry the disease-causing spirochete, *Borrelia burgdorferi,* the agent that causes Lyme disease. Only a relatively low percentage of ticks are infected with *B. burgdorferi*. Blacklegged ticks can also transmit one type

> *Only in America…do we use the word politics to describe the process so well: 'Poli' in Latin means 'many' and 'tics' meaning 'bloodsucking creatures'.*
> —Anonymous

> **Fact:** *In order to transmit a tick-borne infection, the tick needs to remain attached to the host for at least 24 to 36 hours.*

of ehrlichiosis, a recently recognized illness that can be rapidly fatal if it is not diagnosed and treated promptly. Blacklegged ticks also carry Babesiosis (caused by the pathogen *Babesia microti.*) What is babesiosis you might ask? It is a parasitic disease characterized by headache, malaise, and fever. Actually headache, malaise, and fever characterize *all* tick-borne diseases, so it's a fairly generic presentation. Can you acquire more than one infection from one tick bite? Unfortunately the answer is yes, although this is an uncommon occurrence.

A second type of ehrlichiosis (known as human granulocytic ehrlichiosis) is spread by the American dog tick (*Dermacentor variabilis*) and, in the South, by the lone star tick, *Amblyomma americanum.* The American dog tick (*Dermacentor variabilis)* also carries Rocky Mountain Spotted Fever, as does the wood tick (*Dermacentor andersoni).*

Diagnosis of tick-borne illnesses. The diagnosis is rather tough to make unless a tick the size of Texas is yanked snatched off the body and is presented to the health care practitioner in its entirety. And, that doesn't happen very often. But, if it does happen, and you find a tick on your body, remove it, throw it into a zip lock bag and bring it in for a thorough examination.

"Tickacillin." Doxycycline hyclate has become an important, empiric, all-purpose "Tickacillin" since it covers both old tick-borne entities such as Rocky Mountain Spotted Fever and Lyme disease as well as the newer tick-borne illnesses such as ehrlichiosis.

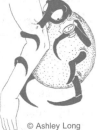
© Ashley Long

Global warming and infectious diseases around the world. Looks like global warming is wreaking havoc within the world of infectious disease. A major 2-year study by the National Center for Ecological Analysis and Synthesis was the first comprehensive effort to analyze epidemics across whole plant and animal systems on land and in the sea.

> ## How to Remove a Tick
>
> If you find a tick attached to the skin, use a pair of narrow-nosed tweezers to grasp the mouthparts as close to the skin as possible. Gently and repeatedly twist the tweezers slowly and steadily and pull straight back. Don't squeeze the tick with the tweezers. Don't use alcohol, Vaseline, nail polish, mouthwash, hot oil, burning matches or other methods sometimes advocated to dislodge ticks. Don't touch the tick or any fluid from the tick. Once the tick has been removed wash the area around the bite wound with an antiseptic. Remember, if you remove a tick within 24 to 36 hours it is extremely unlikely to transmit an infection. Unlike mosquitoes, ticks are slow eaters and spend many hours injecting an array of chemicals to prepare their feeding site. *(AFP 2002;66;643-5)*

Researchers found that climate-related outbreaks are occurring in a wide range of hosts, including corals, birds, oysters, plants, and humans. Even slight increases in temperature allow disease-causing viruses, bacteria and fungi to develop more rapidly. As global temperatures rise, these carriers spread into new areas that were previously inhospitable. For example, insects carrying tropical diseases are heading toward the poles. Cold weather has often been the principal check on these germs; with shorter, milder winters, more of them are surviving. These changes could lead to the extinction of species and cause more illness in humans. "It's not only going to be a warmer world, it's going to be a sicker world," says epidemiologist Andrew Dobson. (*Science*, July 7, 2002)

Global warming and health issues. Diseases carried by the mosquito will be moving north as the climate warms up. Mosquito-borne infections will become more prevalent because their insect carriers, also known as "vectors," are very sensitive to meteorological conditions. For my faithful subscribers in the South, the same faithful subscribers who give me grief for living in Chicago, take heed—*cold can be a friend to humans.* Cold weather limits mosquitoes to seasons and regions where temperatures stay above certain minimums. Winter freezing kills many eggs, larvae, and adult mosquitoes outright.

The *Anopheles* mosquitoes, the vector for malaria parasites (such as *Plasmodium faciparum*), cause sustained outbreaks for malaria only where temperatures routinely exceed 60° F (15.5° C). The *Aedes aegypti* mosquitoes, the vectors responsible for yellow fever and dengue fever, convey the virus only where temperatures rarely fall below 50° F (10° C).

Since 1990, when the hottest decade on record in the U.S. began, outbreaks of locally transmitted malaria have occurred in Texas, Florida, Georgia, Michigan, New York, and New Jersey. Most likely a stow-away mosquito carrying the malaria parasite from a traveler to Africa or Asia was the culprit. Apparently the malaria parasite found the U.S. not only to be a parasite-friendly, warm and cuddly, humid place, but it also found enough mosquitoes able to transport them to victims who had *not* traveled to far away places with strange-sounding names.

Mosquitoes and replication times. Mosquitoes infect over 700 million people throughout the world every year. As the air becomes warmer, mosquitoes proliferate faster and bite more. Heat also speeds the rate at which pathogens inside the mosquito reproduce and mature. For example, the immature malaria parasite, *P. falciparum,* takes 28 days to mature in 68° F (20° C) weather. Bump up that outdoor thermostat to 77° F (25° C) and it only takes 13 days to fully mature. Since the mosquito that spreads the malaria parasite only lives a few weeks, warmer temperatures boost the probability that the malaria parasite will mature in time for the mosquito to transmit the infection.

The deforestation and doubling of some African populations every 20 years has resulted in more people living near areas favorable for breeding mosquitoes. From 1970 to 1990, malaria incidence in Rwanda increased eightfold. Malaria kills about 2.7 million people each year.

QUICK BITE: The average mosquito consumes around one millionth of a gallon of blood per "bite." At that rate, it would take somewhere around 1,120,000 bites to drain the blood from an average adult human. (*The Mosquito Book,* 1998)

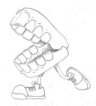

© Ashley Long

The mosquito bite. Only the female bites. She bites to provide nutrition to develop her eggs, not to provide nutrition for her own physiologic needs. The nutritional needs of mosquitoes are met primarily by flower nectar and sugars from rotting fruit.

Less than 5 percent of our skin contains blood vessels or capillaries, therefore mosquitoes have to plunge their proboscis up and down, down and up, back and forth, and forth and back numerous times (as many as 20 times) in order to hit the blood vessel bingo. By the way, she prefers venules (small veins) and arterioles (small arteries) as compared to capillaries (small connecting vessels)—more pressure, faster fill-up time. The mosquito will focus on a specific area for approximately ten seconds at a time and, if the first plunge is un-"suck"cessful, so to speak, she withdraws her blood-seeking proboscis and dives into an adjacent patch of skin. Once she strikes blood, she frantically sucks two to three times her body weight in blood in ninety seconds—keeping one eye out for the big SWAT that might interrupt her feeding at any given moment. The amount consumed is tantamount to a 150-pound human consuming 300-450 pounds of food at the Old Country Buffet. We're talkin' stuffed here—uncomfortable-stuffed, loosening-the-belt buckle-stuffed, pushing-back-from-the-table-stuffed, moaning and groaning-stuffed, declaring that you'll never-eat-another-bite-stuffed. Sound familiar?

Can a mosquito burst from eating too much? Actually, the answer is no. The female stops feeding once stretch receptors in her abdomen have been stimulated. This sends a message to the brain that halts the meal. However, experimentally, if the nerves connecting the abdominal stretch receptors to the brain are cut, the female will suck blood until she bursts.

Of course, after consuming two to three times one's body weight at a single meal, it is understandable that there would be a sense of fullness accompanied by a pervasive sense of sluggishness. Bloated mosquitoes are not the quickest sprinter out of the gate, so to speak, therefore they can barely move to a quiet place to lie low while they digest. They will literally fly away and hit the closest vertical surface, a wall, a post, or a tree trunk for their after-the-meal siesta. The next 45 minutes is critical to the survival of the developing mosquito larvae.

As mom relaxes after the mega-meal, her digestive system draws water out of the blood just consumed and excretes it in the form of "mosquito urine." You, as the "bitee," may actually observe this process after you have served as her supper. The "mosquito urine" is secreted as a pink-tinged fluid dripping out of her anus. Too much information? Anyway, she subsequently stores the remainder of the meal in order to feed her developing offspring.

Your reward for serving as her main meal is an itchy, scratchy, wheal that is irritating to say the least. Substances in her saliva cause the release of histamine and other substances from your cells causing a local reaction known as a mosquito bite, or in some unlucky individuals the histamine is released in all tissues and causes a systemic reaction known as anaphylaxis.

Why do some of us have all the luck when it comes to providing a feeding frenzy for an expectant mother mosquito? Do mosquitoes like the outfit you're wearing? Do they like the smell of your breath? Your body odor? The smell of your feet? Apparently, the answer is all of the above. They like dark colored clothing, "ox" breath, and "limburger cheese" feet. Let me explain.

CO_2 (carbon dioxide) receptors located on their "palpi" (little facial feelers), can detect a whiff of the gas at a distance of 50 to 100 feet. In other words, mosquitoes are waiting for *you* to exhale. In addition to CO_2, mosquitoes are attracted to lactic acid, secreted via the skin and breath. Every individual has varying amounts of lactic acid—helping to explain why some of us are more attractive dining companions for the female mosquito. It seems as if men have more than women and adults have more than children.

Another body chemical that serves as a mosquito pheromone is octanol, a substance first discovered in the breath of an ox that is produced by grass fermenting in the stomach. The corollary here would be any human having ox breath has a better chance of being on the receiving end of the mosquito feeding frenzy. Actually, eating too many green leafy vegetables may increase your susceptibility by making your skin and breath ooze more octanol. SonicWeb is a new contraption that supposedly attracts mosquitoes *away* from living, breathing mammals. It has an audible heartbeat, gives off a small amount of heat and the clincher—it emits an odor that smells just like ox breath. Visit *www.sonicweb.com* for more information on this bug-bashing, mosquito-mangling machine.

Now, here is the explanation for the mosquito affinity for feet that smell like Limburger cheese. A bit of history is necessary: Odor-producing bacteria generally inhabit smelly feet and smelly cheese. In fact, bacteria are essential in the production of smelly cheeses, and it has been suggested by some historians that certain bacteria involved in cheese production actually originated from the feet of Belgian monks—the inventors of Limburger cheese, the smelliest cheese of all.

Let's return to the original story. Researchers placed mosquitoes in a small wind tunnel with two traps, one trap with Limburger fumes and the other trap with good old fresh clean air. The mosquitoes, *Anopheles gambiae* made a buzz line directly to the cheese trap, bypassing the fresh clean air with nary a nod in that direction. The second part of the experiment involved a room full of male volunteers scantily clad in Superman briefs. The mosquitoes were let loose in the room and headed directly for the ankles and feet, biting furiously and leaving the remainder of the body bite-free. The final step in the research project was the coup d'état. The volunteers scrubbed their feet and ankles with antibacterial soap. The unsuspecting *Anopheles gambiae* were appalled and would have absolutely nothing to do with the freshly scrubbed feet.

Do mosquitoes just bite humans? No, and, as a matter of fact, humans are not their first choice for a meal. Most species of mosquitoes prefer birds. Remember that the mosquito dines on blood for the sole purpose of providing an essential protein for the development of the mosquito eggs. That protein just happens

> *Mosquitoes cannot transmit the human immunodeficiency virus (HIV) that causes AIDS, because HIV does not survive in the mosquito gut. Even if it could, the viral concentration in most HIV-infected persons is so low that the odds against it being transmitted by a mosquito bite are estimated at less than 1 in 10 million.*
> (Washington Post/Health/ July 28, 1998)

to be the amino acid isoleucine. Isoleucine is found in much greater concentrations in the blood of birds as compared to the capillaries of your feet, but since we make a bigger target, and we also have smelly breath and feet, and we're not as much of a moving target we tend to be the easier meal of choice. Mosquitoes will also bite just about anything, including snakes and frogs.

How do mosquitoes transmit disease? Before sucking your blood, the female mosquito injects her saliva, which contains an anticoagulant as well as a protein that causes the "bump." This is also how she transmits the many pathogens (viruses, parasites) that cause over 100 diseases.

Historical Highlights

Yellow fever. 'Twas the summer of 1793, in the nation's capital of Philadelphia, Pennsylvania, when yellow fever wiped out one-tenth of the population of 50,000. The trigger for the epidemic appeared to be the arrival of refugees from Saint Domingue (the island known today as Haiti). The refugees landed on the banks of the Delaware River, on the east side of the city. They described a mysterious fever that decimated the population of several islands in the West Indies.

Shortly after their arrival, in July 1793, a similar fever struck the Philadelphia residents living along the Delaware River where the refugees landed. In addition to the high fevers, their eyes and skin turned yellow and they died from internal bleeding within days of becoming ill. By August 19, a prominent Philadelphia physician had given the disease a name—"bilious remitting yellow fever." And, more importantly, he warned the existing government that an epidemic was imminent. By August 26 the College of Physicians recommended specific public health measures to combat and contain the epidemic.

Since infectious disease had not yet become a subspecialty in the world of medicine in the eighteenth century, the prevailing theory of disease centered around the spread of disease by the putrid vapors of decaying vegetable matter and animal carcasses that were rotting in the streets. In addition, fluids and other "vapors" given off by the patient were also blamed for the spread of the disease. It didn't seem to cross anyone's mind that the open sewers, the rotting food and animal carcasses

Mosquito bites. Adults say they average 10 mosquito bites per week during mosquito season. They claim to get the most mosquito bites in July (49 percent), August (29 percent), June (13 percent), September (5 percent), and May (4 percent). (Impulse Research Corporation for OFF! Mosquito Lamp)

Antibiotic use in animals and subsequent human resistance. More than 80 percent of the infections with *Salmonella* and *Campylobacter* in humans are acquired from animals eaten as food. The unfortunate news is that many of those strains of bacteria are resistant to antibiotics. How did this resistance happen? The antibiotics used in humans (tetra-

lining the major thoroughfares, as well as the outhouses might have something to do with disease transmission. In fact, the physicians attributed the "bilious remitting yellow fever" to a spoiled shipload of coffee that arrived at the same time the refugees arrived from the West Indies.

The public health measures that were instituted included avoiding those who were ill and covering the mouth and nose with cloths soaked with camphor and vinegar. In addition, gunpowder was burned to clear the air. The city also started to reinforce the laws mandating bi-weekly trash pick-ups, along with picking up the dead carcasses and rotting vegetables. And, the College of Physicians recommended that the mayor of Philadelphia ban the ringing of church funeral bells, which had been ringing nonstop to announce the many deaths in the city.

Little did anyone know that this "bilious remitting yellow fever" was a viral infection carried in the female mosquito of the species known as *Aedes aegypti.* The mosquito had hopped on the boats carrying the refugees from Saint Domingue to the east banks of the Delaware River in Philadelphia. Mosquitoes that were infected with the virus bit the unsuspecting adult and transmitted the virus during their feeding frenzy.

It wasn't until 107 years later that Dr. Walter Reed proved the theory that yellow fever was transmitted to humans via the mosquito bite.

> *The Surgeon General of the United States Army has approved the report of a special medical board, which has reached the conclusion that the mosquito is responsible for the transmission of yellow fever. The medical department is moving energetically to put into practical operation the methods of treatment for prevention of yellow fever. The liberal use of coal oil to prevent the hatching of mosquito eggs is recommended.*
>
> (*U.S. Army bacteriologist Walter Reed submitted the report.*)

cycline, penicillin, sulfonamides, and the fluoroquinolones) are also given to the pigs, cows, and chickens that end up on the dinner table. Animals are routinely given low doses of these antibiotics in feed and water to act as growth promoters and to prevent illness. The Animal Health Institute defends the practice and points out that animals given low levels of antibiotics grow fatter more quickly and stay healthy longer than those not on antibiotics. It is estimated that 27.6 million pounds of antibiotics are given to animals each year to promote growth. And, oh by the way, antibiotics are also used for infections in the animals as well. (See chicken "snickering" next page.)

A popular misconception about antibiotics and meat and poultry is that the antibiotic remains in the meat in large quantities. Not true. The FDA requires that livestock operators withdraw antibiotics for a certain period of time prior to slaughter; therefore, antibiotic residues are rarely a problem. Although meat and poultry contain antibiotic-resistant bacteria, proper cooking and handling kills even superbugs.

Fighting Flora with Flora—Preempt. Preempt, a mixture containing the normal flora of the gut of healthy chickens, has been ap-

def'i·ni'tions

Malaria. Malaria is the combination of two Italian words—"mala" meaning "bad" and "aria" meaning "air." This expression was used in the eighteenth century by the European settlers in Africa who believed that this disease was from noxious air emanating from the swamplands of Africa. They were kind of right. The swamps were the source of mosquitoes that carried the parasite; however, they thought that it was the "vapors" from the swamplands that caused the disease. The Europeans decided to move to the mountainous areas of Africa to escape the bad air.

proved by the FDA (1998) to spray on chicks as soon as they hatch. The mixture contains 29 benign bacterial species and helps prevent colonization of the chicks by *Salmonella*, and will also perhaps prevent *E. Coli O157:H7, Listeria,* and *Campylobacter jejuni. Salmonella* has reached epidemic proportions in the U.S. It is responsible for 2 to 4 million cases of human illness per year. The Preempt mixture of healthy bacteria works by binding to all of the available sites in the intestines where *Salmonella* might otherwise bind. This strategy is known as "competitive exclusion."

This strategy basically mimics what mother hens naturally do for their baby chicks. The hens pass their own intestinal flora to their offspring when the young chicks peck at their fecal droppings. In our modern-day chicken-producing methods, baby hatchlings are separated from their mother hens at birth and are subsequently prevented from acquiring the normal flora that prevents *Salmonella* binding. They are thus susceptible to colonization with pathogenic bacterial flora. (Stephenson, J. Fighting flora with flora: FDA approves an anti-*Salmonella* spray for chickens. *JAMA 1998*: (279): 1152)

The case of the chicken "snickering." If a poultry farmer notices that a few of the baby chickens, also known as hatchlings, (why aren't they called chicklets?) in the "grow-out" building have started snickering (the

A glass of milk may contain miniscule amounts of up to 80 different antibiotics.

def'i·ni'tions

Sepsis. The word sepsis comes from the Greek word meaning "to putrefy". In the early 1800's sepsis was thought to be a kind of combustion caused by exposing moist body tissues to oxygen.

equivalent of coughing in the world of chickens), he will immediately treat the entire grow-out building within 72 hours. The snickering is often the first sign of an upper respiratory infection and it could spread to all 20,000 hatchings in less than three days. So, the veterinarian recommends enrofloxacin, the animal version of the human antibiotic ciprofloxacin, also known as "Cipro." Since it is almost impossible to isolate the few hatchlings that are the "snickerers," the poultry farmer will just dump five gallons of enrofloxacin in the drinking water of the entire grow-out building. One week later, nary a snicker is heard. Twenty thousand chickens have been saved, so to speak, only to meet their demise at the guillotine six weeks later.

The good news. Enrofloxacin kills the respiratory bug and saves the flock.

The bad news. Enrofloxacin allows the gastrointestinal bug, *Campylobacter jejuni* to flourish and to develop resistance to the human version ciprofloxacin. The chickens develop drug resistance genes that are spread to the rest of the flock. Once destroyed and carved up in the slaughterhouse, the pathogens are spread throughout the place—even with the best sanitary controls. *C. jejuni* is shrunk-wrapped right along with your favorite thigh, wing, or breast, and delivered directly to the consumer. Hence, drug resistance to ciprofloxacin is becoming more prevalent and is just the tip of the proverbial iceberg when it comes to antibiotic resistance.

Smelly feet. The moist foot is a haven for bacteria. The wetter the foot or shoe, the more at home the bacteria will feel. The moist foot can harbor up to 6 trillion bacteria—the dry foot, zero.

How should you keep your feet dry? Spray the same antiperspirant on your feet

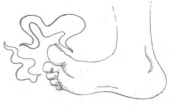

© Ashley Long

that you douse your underarms with. Feet actually have more sweat glands than your armpits so a healthy dose of antiperspirant (especially one that contains aluminum chlorhydrate) will help to partially block the sweat glands and ducts. Take an extra pair of socks or hose to the office and change them during the day. Don't wear the same pair of shoes two days in a row. Give the shoes 24 hours to "breathe," dry out, and recover after a day wrapped around your smelly, damp feet.

Well, what if that doesn't work? Steep three tea bags in a pint of water and then let the water cool. Soak the soles of both feet for 20 minutes at least three times per week for two weeks. After two weeks, repeat the process once a week or so. The tannic acid in the tea stimulates the proteins in the epidermis to "stick together." This thickens the soles of the feet and helps to block the sweat glands and ducts. The feet are drier, bacteria are depressed, and they move on to the next unsuspecting "sole" in Nikes.

E. Coli O157:H7 produces the third most deadly toxin in the world. Tetanus and botulinum toxin (the agent of botulism) are the first two on the list. The amount of *E. Coli O157:H7* bacteria that can make you sick is only 10 to 100 pathogens. If you are immunocompromised, very young, or very old, this amount of pathogen can actually not just make you sick, it can kill you.

E.Coli was discovered in 1885 by a German pediatrician Theodor Escherich. He initially named the pathogen Bacterium coli commune; however, in 1919 the name was changed to honor the discoverer, *Escherichia Coli,* or *E. Coli.*

In the Spring of 2001 a New York City man was arrested for spraying feces-laden water over the contents of a midtown Manhattan salad bar. Fortunately, it was your everyday run-of-the-mill *E.Coli* found in human feces, not the virulent strain *E.Coli O157:H7* that inhabits the intestinal tract of 23 to 28 percent of the cattle in this country.

Patients have been known to infect their own wounds with feces or to inject feces into their own IV lines to cause illness and a temperature spike. These patients have Munchausen's syndrome. Munchausen syndrome patients actually fake their illnesses by describing or creating unusual and perplexing patterns of symptoms. For example, they may take massive quantities of unrelated medications; they may inject themselves with urine or feces; they may deposit blood or feces in samples of their own urine submitted for laboratory tests.

A controversial eponym. Hans Conrad Julius Reiter, a German physician (1881-1969) first reported a case of Reiter's syndrome in 1916. Even though Reiter first reported the syndrome in 1916 the eponym was adapted by the English language journals in the early 1940s. He described a condition of systemic inflammation "that appears to be an immunologic reaction to a sexually transmitted infection or dysentery to people who have a genetic predisposition to it." This syndrome is associated with urethritis (inflammation of the urethra), arthritis (inflammation of the joints), and conjunctivitis (inflammation of the conjunctiva of the eye). *Chlamydia trachomatis* is the organism most frequently associated with Reiter's syndrome.

The controversy....Dr. Hans Reiter was an early disciple of Adolph Hitler and evidence continues to accumulate concerning Dr. Reiter's role in planning and approving "human experiments" in German concentration camps. As President of the Reich Health Office in 1937, Dr. Reiter was a proponent of the Nazi belief that inferior genes should not be transmitted. Dr. Reiter sanctioned experiments that killed thousands of concentration camp prisoners. He "devised orders, supervised medical atrocities and gave the stamp of approval for them." In one Reiter-approved experiment, 250 prisoners at Buchenwald died after they were purposefully infected with *rickettsia*.

As a result of his involvement in the atrocities of Hitler's regime, calls are being made to remove his name from this syndrome. In fact, the Spondylitis Association of America, a patient advocacy group that represents people with Reiter's syndrome, recently voted to call Reiter's syndrome reactive arthritis, dropping the eponym once and for all. It remains to be seen as to whether authors, editors and other medical leaders will do the same for future textbooks and articles.

Infection control imponderables. (Schweon, SJ. *Journal of Nursing Jocularity 1998; 6 (3)*.)

• Why are electric chairs cleansed and disinfected between electrocutions?

• Why, before a lethal injection is administered in prison, is the skin prepped with alcohol to prevent infection?

The perils of pedicures. Keep an eye on the feet of your patients who use the whirlpool footbaths for pedicures at the local nail salons. These are breeding grounds for pesky pathogens that can cause serious bacterial skin infections if the baths aren't properly cleaned. This is particularly true if the individual has shaved her legs prior to plopping her feet into the whirlpool, since shaving makes it easier for the bacteria to enter the skin. More than 100 customers developed multiple boils and skin ulcers after using an inadequately cleaned whirlpool in a Watsonville, California salon. Unfortunately many of the cases left unsightly scars on the lower legs of the customers. And the pathogens were primarily antibiotic-resistant bugs. Most states require that the foot basins be rinsed and disinfected between customers (that's reassuring); however, some states don't require cleaning the filter that traps skin and hair. Customers can protect themselves by calling the salon prior stopping by, checking the salon's business license, inquiring about disinfection practices, and refraining from shaving before the procedure. (*New Engl J Med,* July 12, 2002*)*

Mad cow disease. This devastating neurological deterioration is fatal in all cases—whether you are a sheep, a cow, a cannibal, or a human with non-cannibalistic preferences. In sheep the disease is known as scrapie (SCRAY-pee), in cows it is known as bovine spongioform encephalopathy (BSE), in the Fore cannibal tribe of New Guinea it is known as kuru, and in non-cannibalistic humans it is referred to as Creutzfeldt-Jakob disease (CJD) or *variant* Creutzfeldt-Jakob disease (vCJD).

The first cases of "mad cow" disease appeared in Britain in 1987. Cows were observed to be disoriented, irritable, apprehensive and unable to stand or walk without a staggering,

> *Do you know why they call it PMS? Because "Mad Cow Disease" was taken.*
> —Unknown, presumed deceased

unsteady gait. Autopsies on the bovine brain revealed "spongy" areas and the name bovine spongioform encephalopathy was given to this disease in cattle. The autopsy findings were similar to those seen in humans dying of CJD and in sheep dying of scrapie. (The term scrapie originates from the behavior of sheep with this illness. The disoriented, demented sheep stand next to the barn or fence and scrape their flank against it until it bleeds.)

In 1996, the first ten British citizens were diagnosed with "mad cow" disease. Since the brain tissue resembled that of the "mad cows" and that of humans dying of CJD, the Bitish pathologists named it *variant* CJD (vCJD). Since 1996, over 85 British citizens have died from vCJD and over 100 have died throughout the European nations. Italy, Germany, France, Spain, Ireland, Belgium, Denmark, Luxembourg, the Netherlands, Switzerland, and Liechtenstein (where?) have all reported cattle infected with mad cow disease.

The cause of BSE is a mutant prion (PREE-on). This is not a virus, parasite, bacteria, fungus, or any other type of infectious agent. The brains of all mammals (and that includes us humans) contain structural proteins in the brain known as prions. Something causes the prion to undergo a structural "unfolding," which in turn acts as somewhat of a toxin causing the surrounding brain tissue to degenerate. Once the prion changes shape the process is a progressive, unremitting, rapid deterioration of mental and motor function.

The exact trigger for the unfolding of the prion is unknown; however, it is most likely triggered by eating brain or spinal cord tissue from another infected animal. Eating cattle infected with the mutant prion caused the vCJD in Erope. The cattle were infected by eating rendered meat-and-bone meal protein supplements made from sheep, cows, pigs, poultry, road kill, and anything other dead animal that happened upon the rendering machine. (Rendering, by the way, means to boil and grind up carcasses of dead animals—including bones, brains, spinal cords, and internal organs.) Most likely the culprit was from renderings of sheep with scrapie and other cattle with BSE.

Notice that the above list of countries did *not* include the U.S. No cases of infected cattle or human forms of vCJD have been diagnosed in the U.S. and hopefully it will stay that way. Our FDA, USDA, and every other regulating agency have their hands in the pot on this one, and safeguards have been put into place. First of all, the USDA banned the importation of sheep and goats to the U.S. as far back as 1950 after a flock of British sheep were reported to have scrapie. They also banned their rumination by-products. The importation of cattle from England was banned in 1989. Fewer than 500 cows from the British Isles made it across the Atlantic Ocean in the 1980s. Of those 500, only 32 entered the food chain. The chance that even one cow was infected is one in 10 billion.

Secondly, the FDA has prohibited animal-feed mills from mixing meat-and-bone meal made from rendered cows and sheep into feed for cows and sheep. The supplements can be fed to swine and poultry, however, because they do not get BSE-like illnesses from food.

The third reason it will be tough for BSE to make its way into our food chain is because of good old McDonald's. Even though they are killing us with the fries and burgers in one way or another, they are adamant that their hamburger source is free of contamination. And, when McDonalds talks, *everyone* listens. McDonald's rules the roost when it comes to beef sales throughout the world. If Mickey D's says that all cattle used for its all-beef patties should have documentation that they have not been fed meat-and-bone meal made from cows and sheep, then by cracky, it's a mandate.

Lastly, the beef industry stopped using stun guns to prepare cattle for the slaughterhouse. The explosive blast from the stun gun blew brain tissue throughout the carcass, causing a potential route of infection with prions in nervous system tissue. In cows with BSE, brain tissue is highly infectious.

Hmmmm, you say. If people didn't eat cow brains or spinal cords, how did they acquire this illness? Most likely from eating inexpensive beef products that contained mechanically separated meat. This type of meat is a paste produced by compressing carcasses. This paste may have contained spinal cords, and was used in preparing hot dogs, sausages, and burgers. Do we use mechanically separated meat in the U.S.? Yes, but rarely. And, the label on the package must state that it includes mechanically separated beef. Unfortunately, there are no labels on hot dogs purchased from hot dog stands or sausages as a side order at you favorite breakfast establishment.

FACT: *In January 2001 the USDA recommended that anyone who had lived in France, Portugal, or Ireland for a total of 10 years since 1980 be prohibited from donating blood. The year before, the USDA recommended a similar exclusion for anyone living in Britain for six months between 1980 and 1996. The interesting point to the blood donor recommendation is that there is absolutely no evidence that the disease can be transmitted through a blood transfusion in the first place. Better to be safe than sorry, I suppose.*

So, is a filet mignon safe? Yes. How about a good old hot dog at Wrigley Field? Yes. How about a good old hot dog in jolly old England? Well, maybe. The European Union has banned mechanically separated beef and that ban has been in full effect since the end of 2001.

Can vegetarians acquire vCJD? Yes, and they have. Most likely their exposure was through milk or gelatin, which is made from beef. Or, vCJD may incubate for decades (the incubation period is unknown at this time), and the vegetarian may have eaten infected beef in the years prior to becoming a vegetarian.

What are the safest cuts of meat? Boneless steaks such as filet mignon, roasts, or other whole cuts of beef are the safest. T-bone, porterhouse, standing rib roast, prime rib with bone, and bone-in chuck blade roast may contain spinal cord tissue or small groups of nerves that line the spinal cord known as dorsal root ganglia, which are infectious if they come from an infected cow.

For more information on CJD, vCJD, BSE, scrapie and kuru, log on to *www.mad-cow.org* or *www.cdc.gov.*

Squirrel brains: a deadly delicacy? Mad cow disease is one of a family of transmissible spongioform encephalopathies that include scrapie in sheep and goats, chronic wasting disease in North American deer and elk, and transmissible mink encephalopathy. We must now consider adding to the list squirrel brains. An article in the July 17, 2000 *New Yorker* describes five patients with Creutzfeldt-Jakob disease (CJD), of which mad cow disease is a variant. All five patients had one thing in common—they ate squirrel brains as a delicacy. Over 25 million squirrels are killed and consumed each year in Kentucky, Ohio, and Tennessee (not to mention Arkansas). An editorial in *The Lancet* (1997; 350 (9078): 642) documents a possible link between CJD and the consumption of squirrel brains.

Reptiles and *salmonella*. Reptiles account for 93,000 cases of *salmonella* per year in the U.S. The sale of small turtles was banned in 1975; however, lizards and snakes are well-known carriers of the bacteria. The iguana has become one of the major carriers now that the turtle has been banned from crossing the border. U.S. imports of iguanas rose from 27,806 in 1986 to an all-time high of 798,405 in 1995. The CDC now recommends that all types of lizards, snakes and turtles should not be household pets, especially if there is a child under the age of five living in the house. The reptiles carry *salmonella* in their GI tract and frequently shed the bug in their feces. Touching the reptile isn't necessary for infection however. Some cases of reptile-associated *salmonella* have occurred in infants who have never handled the scaly creatures; however, the pet owners have handled the infant with pet fecal matter on their hands. There is no reliable test or treatment to ensure that a pet reptile won't carry the bacteria.

Saliva as a defense mechanism. Saliva, one of the body's innate barrier defense mechanisms, has antimicrobial proteins as well as protective secretory antibodies known as IgA. These natural protective effects help to explain why sexually transmitted diseases such as HIV are not easily transmitted by kissing or by dental procedures.

A new finding provides an additional protective property of saliva—the lack of significant amounts of salt. In fact, saliva has one-seventh the amount of salt as other body fluids. When pathogens are placed in a salt-free environment, the intracellular concentration of salt in the pathogen provides a strong osmotic "pull" from the water-based saliva. Water enters the pathogen causing the cell to literally "blow-up" from the water overload.

On the other hand, saliva *doesn't* protect during oral sex or breast-feeding. The addition of saltier fluids from either of those activities counterbalances saliva's low salinity. (*Archives of Internal Medicine,* March 1999)

Sea otters and kitty litter. It appears as if kitty feces, infected with *Toxoplasma gondii,* may be partially responsible for the decline in the sea otter population along the California coastline. Dr. Melissa Miller, wildlife veterinarian, tested 223 live and dead sea otters for these parasites that are excreted in feral cat and opposum feces. Miller found that 42 percent of the live sea otters and 62 percent of the dead sea otters carried antibodies (signifying an immune response) to the pathogen. Kitty feces, from storm-drain runoff may carry the parasites to the ocean where they come into contact with the sea otters. Sea otters live right along the coastline near sites of freshwater runoff—rivers and streams that carry untreated water from fields and yards into the ocean. The sea otters are acquiring *Toxoplasma gondii* by swallowing seawater or by eating sandcrabs contaminated with the pathogen. Only 2,000 of the California sea otters remain along the California coastline.

Strep infections, toothbrushes and dental appliances. Perhaps little Petunia's persistent strep throat has nothing to do with her being a strep carrier and everything to do with her toothbrush harboring the strep bacteria. A study published in the February 24, 1999 issue of *JAMA* found that strep organisms from throat infections could be cultured from toothbrushes as well as from orthodontic appliances. In patients who tested positive for strep throats, cultures were also taken from their toothbrushes and orthodontic devices before and after a 10-day course of penicillin. Even after treatment had ended, 17 percent of the throats continued to test positive for the strep. Strep was found in 28 percent of the toothbrushes and 19 percent of the orthodontic devices cultured.

Twenty of the positive toothbrushes were divided into two groups, ten in each group. In the ten that were rinsed daily, the strep bug disappeared within three days. However, in the ten that were not rinsed daily, the strep persisted for up to 15 days. The moral of the story is rather obvious. Advise patients who are being treated for strep to thoroughly rinse their toothbrushes and orthodontic appliances each time they brush.

Strep infections and Tourette's syndrome. A possible trigger for Tourette's syndrome is a strep infection caused by group A Beta Hemolytic Strep (GABHS). Tourette's syndrome runs in families, however it manifests in only a small number of children inheriting the gene. A cross-reaction with the GABHS antigens results in the immune system producing antibodies against neurons in one of the movement areas of the brain known as the basal ganglia. This is the area of the brain responsible for the control of involuntary movements such as tics and involuntary cursing outbursts known as corprolalia. (Singer, H. Johns Hopkins' University, Department of Neurology)

Sushi and infections. Skip the salmon sushi if you want to enjoy raw fish at your local Japanese restaurant. Federal investigators tested fish in 32 Seattle-area sushi bars and found that servings of uncooked salmon (called *sake*) were infected one in ten times with roundworms that can cause illness in people. Raw tuna (called *maguro*), the most popular kind of sushi, wasn't a problem. (*Health*, March/April 1995)

Swimming and the plague. Swimming was eschewed in Europe during the Middle Ages, because outdoor bathing was mistakenly cited as a cause of spreading epidemics and plagues that periodically ravaged the continent. It wasn't until the latter portion of the nineteenth century that swimming returned to popularity.

Syphilis and venereal disease, or VD. Venereal disease or VD, is the "old term" for diseases that are transmitted sexually. The term has been changed to protect the not-so-innocent, and is now known as STD, or sexually transmitted disease, or STI, for sexually transmitted infection. Venereal disease was named after the Roman goddess of beauty,

Historical Highlights

Smallpox was first recorded in history over 10,000 years ago. The mummified remains of Ramses V (1156 B.C.) demonstrated smallpox scars. In 569 A.D. a smallpox epidemic struck Arabia and forced the Ethiopian army to retreat thus ending their rule in Arabia. This was known as the Elephant War epidemic, after the white elephant on which the Christian prince Abraha rode into Mecca before his defeat. This was described in the Koran and was one of the earliest recorded epidemics of smallpox.

Early Spanish explorers brought smallpox to the Americas. Some historians give the credit to Hernando Cortés and others give the credit to Christopher Columbus. If Cortés gets the credit, he brought smallpox to the New World circa 1520, however, if Columbus takes the honors, smallpox entered the Americas in 1492. Between 1520 and 1522, 3.5 million Aztecs died of smallpox. Pocahontas died of smallpox after visiting London in 1617. George Washington developed smallpox after visiting Barbados in 1751, but he survived his bout, albeit severely scarred. Smallpox was rampant in Europe during the eighteenth century as well, killing one in seven children in Russia and one in ten children in Sweden and France. Kings and Queens of France, Spain, Austria, Germany, Russia, and England succumbed to smallpox.

One of the first known "bioterrorist" acts with smallpox occurred during the French/Indian War. Jeffery Amherst gave blankets from British smallpox victims to the Indians, resulting in a smallpox epidemic in the Ohio Valley.

Smallpox has killed hundreds of millions of people around the world and as late as 1967 it was still infecting between 10 and 15 million people worldwide and killing more than 2 million. The World Health Organization (WHO) began its 330 million dollar campaign to eradicate smallpox worldwide in 1967. On May 8, 1980 the WHO declared the disease totally eradicated from the world's population. After the World Health Organization declared smallpox to be officially eradicated, they urged all laboratories around the world to consolidate their stocks of virus and transfer them for storage at either the CDC in Atlanta or the Institute of Viral Preparations in Moscow. While everyone was arguing whether or not to destroy all smallpox and therefore eradicate it off the face of the earth, the threat of bioterrorism reared its ugly head.

It is assumed that North Korea, Iraq, and a few other countries have stockpiled smallpox for possible use. It is a known fact (however, no surprise) that Russia violated an international treaty, and produced more than 20 tons of smallpox virus specifically for dissemination via bombs and intercontinental ballistic missiles. And, before we become indignant about Russia not holding up their end of the bargain with the international treaty, let it also be known that our own U.S. Army also violated the same treaty and stockpiled bioweapons in nooks and crannies throughout the U.S.

Tourette's Syndrome
(George Gilles de la Tourette)

CASE STUDY—Perhaps the most famous of all cases of Tourette's syndrome was that of the noblewoman, the Marquise de Dampierre (1799-1884). The Marquise was notorious for blurting out, in public, for no apparent reason, inappropriate or obscene words, with a particular fondness for "merde et foutu cochon," (translation literally meaning "shit and filthy pig," however the more accurate colloquial meaning of "fouton cochon " at the time, was "fucking pig"). As you might surmise, the behavior of the Marquise Dampierre was quite the talk of the town in the socialite circles of Paris for the greater part of the 1800s.

The chief physician at l'Institution Royale des Sourds-muets in Paris, Jean Marc Gaspard Itard, originally reported the tale of the Marquise in 1825. Dr. Itard first saw his patient when she was 26 years of age. His description was published in the *Archives Générales de Médicine* and reads as follows:

"In the midst of a conversation that interests her extremely, all of a sudden, without being able to prevent it, she interrupts what she is saying or what she is listening to with bizarre shouts and with words that are even more extraordinary and which make a deplorable contrast with her intellect and her distinguished manners. These words are for the most part gross swear words and obscene epithets and, something that is no less embarrassing for her than for the listeners, an extremely crude expression of a judgment or of an unfavorable opinion of someone in the group."

Years later, the Marquise was seen by the leading neurologist in France, the distinguished Jean Martin Charcot, chief physician of the Salpêtrière Hospital of Paris. A twenty-eight- year-old protégé of Charcot was primarily working with ticcing patients at the time. Charcot directed him to organize his patients for clinical publication and the young M.D. chose the Marquise de Campierre as the primary example of a patient with the "maladie des tics," as it was called at the time. This young physician was none other than Georges Gilles de la Tourette and his first paper was published in 1885. Right after the paper was published, Dr. Charcot renamed the convulsive tic illness in honor of the author—Gilles de la Tourette. It appears as if this was rather controversial since this malady had been described in numerous textbooks and articles since the original publication by Itard in 1825.

The cause of the Marquise's ticcing was unknown but Itard was convinced that if she became a wife and a mother, her symptoms would disappear. Much to Itard's dismay, when she married her symptoms very quickly reappeared, and he was quick to point out that it was because she had no child and "was deprived of the favorable benefits that the physical and moral revolution ordinarily provided by maternity would have offered her."

love, eros, drink, and every other hedonistic pleasure known to man. We all know this goddess as Venus. Venereal literally means "whatever pertains to the act of love."

Some syphilitic facts on file:

- Howard Hughes, the clean freak "fuhgillionaire," died of neurosyphillis.

- In the sixteenth century the causes of syphilis were hotly debated. They ranged from soldiers dining on human flesh, libidinous males fornicating with a horse's hiney, French lepers sleeping with prostitutes, *and* the most heinous crime of all—gasp!—the wearing of linen shirts.

- Our intelligence quotient didn't improve by leaps and bounds between the sixteenth and the early twentieth century. The American Navy removed *all* doorknobs from the doors in the barracks, convinced that doorknobs were efficient purveyors of syphilis. The question begs to be asked: What were our "seamen" doing with those doorknobs that they weren't sharing with their superior officers?

- The New World gave the Old World the great pox (syphilis), and not to be outdone in the disease-swapping category, the Old World gave the New World smallpox. Such a deal.

- Columbus and his merry band of libidinous sailors first acquired syphilis on the island of Espanola, presently known as Haiti.

- Columbus and his merry band of libidinous sailors sailed from Haiti to Barcelona, Spain, stopping at a few ports along the way. Everywhere they stopped, they left the gift of the great pox for those with whom they slept. In fact, it was an honor *and* a privilege to sleep with one of the crewmen of Columbus' ship.

- One in every five French citizens had the great pox in the seventeenth century. (And who said these were chaste times?)

- Wigs were first worn by aristocrats in sixteenth century France, England, and Scotland, trying to hide the baldheads of the syphilitic nobility. Mary Queen of Scots and Queen Elizabeth I were two famous Queens left hairless by either the disease of syphilis, or its treatment, mercury.

- Others who have gone before us with the badge of the syphilitic baldhead include *Frances I* of France, King Henry the VIII of England, Ivan the Terrible of Russia, and Pope Julius II. (Did I just say the POPE?)

Syphilis as a method of biological warfare. When the English and French troops marched into Madrid in the early eighteenth century, King Philip V of Spain encouraged the city's starving prostitutes to "sleep with the enemy." They did, and half of the British and French Armies developed the great pox. So much for their undying love, devotion and faithfulness to the loved ones left behind.

The syphilitic "short-faced bear." The oldest known mammal with syphilis was found in Fulton County, Indiana in 1993. The victim was a "short-faced bear" (an extinct species) who appeared to have syphilis around 11,500 years ago. The manner in which he contracted the disease will never be known, nor might we ever *want* to know. He could have devoured an infected human; however, the earliest know case of human syphilis was only 5,000 years ago.

Tattoos and infectious disease. Tattooing has been linked to the transmission of numerous infectious diseases, including syphilis, tuberculosis, leprosy, HIV, and Hepatitis C. The results of a recent study

def'i·ni'tions

Haircut. Haircut used to be used as a dialect word for the primary lesion of syphilis. The allusion was to the former medical custom of shaving the pubic hair when applying the topical therapy for this "venereal" disease.

"Hi, Jack!" Hi, Jack! Was the prostitute's greeting to a lonely sailor on shore leave. Distracted by the greeting from the prostitute, the sailor was boinked on the head by her companion and then sold to a ship in need of a crew. Of course, the meaning is slightly different today. The two words have been condensed into one word, hijack, and it means nothing more than the illegal seizure of cargo or a vehicle.

from the University of New Mexico found that 25 of 58 cases of patients with hepatitis C had tattoos and no other risk factors for hepatitis C. These results suggest that more than one-third of the cases of sporadic hepatitis C may be linked to tattooing (at least in New Mexico).

Other communicable diseases associated with body piercing and tattooing include toxic shock syndrome, hepatitis B, tetanus, sporotrichosis, human papilloma virus (HPV), molluscum contagiosum (viral warts), vaccinia, rubella, chancroid, and herpes simplex virus (HSV). (Kenneth Horn, MS, MSN, FNP, University of South Dakota, Student Health Service)

Healing times for site-specific tattoos are as follows:
- Lower ear soft tissue – six weeks
- Eye brow – six weeks
- Nose – six weeks to nine months
- Mouth, tongue, lip – eight weeks
- Nipple – six to eight weeks
- Umbilical (belly button) – greater than six months
- Genitalia – varied healing time starting at four weeks

(Kenneth Horn, see above)

Tattoos and living wills. A 40-year-old licensed practical nurse is quite adamant about *not* being maintained on a life-support system and she wants to make sure that those taking care of her know about it. She has had a living will tattooed to her abdomen for all to read when the time comes to unplug the respirator and take her off all life-support systems.

Tattoo removal. The cost of having a fist-sized tattoo removed 5 years ago was about $10,000 compared to under $500 today. Close to 20 million Americans have a tattoo somewhere on a body part.

Tattoos on "private parts." A tale from the hospital wards is appropriate at this point in time. A big ol' veteran nurse of 32 years huffed and puffed into the nurses' station one morning after all of the baths and clean-ups were given. She was jibber-jabberin' with her colleagues and one of those colleagues was a cute, perky little new graduate with a full head of blonde hair and big blue innocent eyes. So the veteran nurse of

32 years was going on and on about giving a bed bath to a young man in room 126 who had a tattoo on his penis. She was appalled and thoroughly disgusted as she was explaining to the group at the nurses' station that he had a tattoo on his penis. In her high-pitched piercing voice she clearly stated that his tattoo said, " 'Swan', whatever that stands for!" The young, blonde new graduate nurse looked up from her charting and exclaimed "NO! Are you talking about Mr. Drummond in room 1262?" The old battle-axe said "Yes, that very same young man." The blonde nurse stood up and exclaimed "That can't be possible. I gave him a bed bath yesterday and his tattoo said 'Saskatchewan'!"

That of course, is the Canadian version of the tale. The version told in Norfolk, Virginia is slightly different, but has the clearly has the same meaning. Let's pick up the story as the big ol' battleax of a Navy Nurse swoops into the nurses' station after giving a young seaman a bath. In her high-pitched piercing voice she clearly stated that his tattoo said, " 'Little', whatever that stands for!" The young, blonde new graduate nurse looked up from her charting and exclaimed "NO! Are you talking about Seaman Sands in room 1262?" The old battle-axe humpfed, "Yes, that very same young seaman." The blonde nurse stood up with a perplexed look on her face and said, "That can't be possible. I gave him a bath yesterday and his tattoo said 'Little Creek Naval Amphibious Base'!"

Tuberculosis. In 400 B.C. Hippocrates declared tuberculosis as the deadliest of all diseases. He treated his patients with "consumption" with a diet of honey, barley gruel, and wine. Of course, survival rates did not increase with this soothing diet. At least Hippocrates served up a dose of compassion with his barley gruel. Other physicians weren't so compassionate. Treatments included a dose of arsenic, attaching a dead fish to the sufferer's chest, suckling milk from a human breast (wondering about the donor breast here), and exorcism of the evil spirits causing this deadly disease.

Cheerful people, the doctors say, resist disease better than glum ones. In other words, the surly bird catches the germ.
–Unknown

A veritable WHO'S WHO of famous TB patients. The following is a list of famous people who have suffered from "consumption," also known as the White Plague. Those with the asterisk died from the disease. King Tutankhamen* (King Tut—circa 1358-1340 B.C.); Cardinal Richelieu* (1585-1642); François Voltaire (1694-1778); Johan Goethe (1749-1832); Simón Bolivar* (1783-1830); John Keats* (1795-1821); Ralph Waldo Emerson (1803-1882); Elizabeth Barrett Browning* (1806-1861); Edgar Allan Poe* (1809-1849); Frédéric Chopin* (1810-1849); Emily Bronte* (1818-1848); Paul Gauguin (1848-1903); Robert Louis Stevenson (1850-1894); Anton Chekhov* (1860-1904); Eleanor Roosevelt* (1884-1962); D.H.Lawrence* (1885-1930); Eugene O'Neill* (1888-1953); Adolph Hitler (1889-1945); George Orwell* (1903-1950); Vivien Leigh* (1913-1967); Nelson Mandela (1918-).

Tuberculosis and the popularity of linoleum as a floor covering. Between 1900 and 1945, U.S. physicians were convinced that sanatoriums were the only way to treat patients suffering from tuberculosis. In order to keep the "bacillus" at bay, the sanatoriums were designed in what one would refer to as "minimalist" décor. Ceilings lost their moldings, windows lost their ledges, architects lost their creativity, and there was no such occupation as a space designer. Wallpaper was considered to be infused with germs, so drab green paint became the color du jour. It covered the ceilings, the walls, the radiators, and the windowpanes. Linoleum was sold as tuberculocidal flooring. By covering the floors the germs would be prevented from lurking in between the floorboards. Advertising flyers claimed that linoleum was easy to clean—especially those gooey, slimy, gummy, slithering balls of spit. Linoleum rapidly became the floor covering of choice, covering every inch of floor space in sanatoriums and households in the U.S. in the 1920s and 1930s.

Does a common virus cause obesity? Yes, you have now heard it all, and you heard it here first. An infectious agent may be a possible contributor to obesity in a small number of individuals who are overweight. The University of Wisconsin in Madison studied 154 overweight adults and found that 15 percent tested positive for antibodies to AD-36, a human adenovirus, demonstrating that they had been infected with this agent earlier in their life. None of the 45 lean controls tested positive for the virus.

Lab animals injected with the adenovirus AD-36 gained enough weight to be classified as clinically obese. A paradoxical characteristic of the virus is that it appears to cause *low* cholesterol and triglycerides along with obesity. Obese humans with AD-36 follow the same pattern—they also have lower cholesterol and triglycerides than other obese individuals who develop their obesity "the old fashioned way"—too many calories and too little exercise. (*ADVANCE for Nurse Practitioners,* November 1997)

Survival of the fittest. A cold virus can survive for up to three hours on a dry surface, such as a doorknob. Herpes virus can survive for 45 minutes on a toilet seat. The nasty *E.Coli O157:H7* can survive for 60 days on a stainless steel countertop. The tubercle bacillus can survive for months in dried sputum.

Water safety around the world. More people die each year from unsafe water than from all forms of violence, including war. Recent data suggest that waterborne infectious organisms cause billions of diarrhea illnesses worldwide and more than two million diarrhea-related deaths each year—mostly infants and children. More than a billion people (one in every five on Earth) do not have access to safe drinking water. These individuals rely on ponds, streams, and other exposed and untreated sources for their drinking water. The percentage of the population with access to safe water in each of the following countries is as follows:
Ethiopia—18 percent
Sudan—45 percent
Pakistan—56 percent
Mexico—72 percent
USA—99 percent
(Water Quality and Health Council: Chlorine Chemistry Council; Harder, B. A safe solution. *Discover* 2003 (163:136-7)

Don't drink the water on airplanes. As if this is your biggest worry on an airplane, but let's just add it to the list. A couple of *Wall Street Journal* reporters collected samples of water from galley and lavatory taps on 14 different flights going every which way from New York to

London to St. Louis. The samples they obtained were contaminated with *E. Coli, Salmonella,* and *Legionella pneumoniae.* Whoa…They also found maggot eggs on one airline. The reporters said, "Contamination was the rule, not the exception to the rule." So, stick with bottled water every time you fly—no drinking out of the faucet in the bathroom, don't brush your teeth using the bathroom water, and use alcohol gel wipes to clean your hands after using the bathroom on the plane.

SARS (severe acute respiratory syndrome) and the airline industry. The airlines have suffered a deadly blow by the SARS epidemic. The tourism industry, especially to China and other Asian countries, took a nosedive as widespread panic hit the streets. Perhaps only one small smile can be elicited by this new mutation of an old corona virus and the current outbreak in Asia. Hong Kong paid big bucks for a new slogan to lure tourists to their city. The new slogan was just about to be released when the SARS epidemic reared its ugly head. The new slogan, needless to say, has been canned. The slogan was: "Hong Kong—takes your breath away."

Speaking of finding bugs in strange places. A sampling of cultures taken from various surfaces in New York City on a fine summer's day might make you think twice about going out in public—for any reason. And if you do go out, you may want to take a pocketful of those alcohol gels with you to wipe your hands after touching various and sundry "common" areas. Here are some of the findings from the study.

- A culture taken from the back seat of a taxi contained *Streptococcus viridans*, a common mouth germ most likely expelled during a coughing fit.

- A movie theatre seat was swarming with *Staphylococcus aureus* shed from the skin, and group B strep, normally found in the vaginal secretions, and *enterococcus,* a fecal germ found in stool. The next time you snuggle down on a cushy movie theater seat make sure you're not wearing short shorts or a skirt with thong underwear…ick. Long pants should become the movie attire of the twenty-first century—thick, long pants.

- Fecal germs were found on bar stools, head phones, and the armrest of a chair in the corporate cafeteria, and a spotless clean-as-a-whistle appearing glass at an exclusive bar on the Upper East Side of Manhattan.

- A public telephone handset was teeming with *Staphylococcus aureus* and beta-hemolytic *Streptococcus,* the bacteria that has the potential to cause "the flesh-eating disease" known as necrotizing fascitis.

> *Eighty percent of all infections are transmitted by touch. Whoa. Wash those hands.* (Tierno, PM. *The Secret Life of Germs*, 2001)

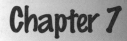

Chapter 7

French Fries & Thunder Thighs

Can vegetarians eat animal crackers?
—Anonymous

Counting calories to lose weight?

• Kissing burns six to twelve calories, depending on the intensity of the kiss. A wild ride in the hay might burn 125 to 300 calories, depending on just how wild that ride gets. If you've been married for 35 years that ride in the hay no longer uses the adjective "wild" and you might burn 125 calories. However, if you have been married only two weeks most likely the encounter will burn at least 300 calories. If you passionately kiss your beloved three times per day and make mad passionate love twice a week, you could theoretically burn 32,000 calories in a year, the equivalent of a 9-pound weight loss. Why are you sitting here reading this book? Don't you have some calories to burn?

- Banging your head against the wall for one hour burns 150 calories. This is the suggested alternative when kissing and mad, passionate lovemaking aren't an option.

- Just eat 100 calories a day more than you expend—like devouring one-half of a Snickers bar—and in 20 years you will gain 100 extra pounds. Ouch. (Dr. Reza Yavari, Endocrinologist, Yale University School of Medicine; *Science Times,* January 15, 2002)

- The average American now eats between 160 to 500 calories more each day than the late 1970s. And we wonder why we're having weight problems? Over a year's time this works out to 270 to 810 extra orders of McDonald's French fries. Americans eat 3.5 metric tons of French fries every year—about 28 pounds per person. (*The Wall Street Journal,* April 2002.)

- Food companies produce 3,800 calories of food a day for every American. In 1970 that number was 3,300 calories for every American. By now you have realized that the difference is 500 calories a day.

- Every second in the U.S. Americans eat 350 slices of pizza. And we wonder why we're having weight problems?

- It takes 3,500 *extra* calories to gain one pound. It takes 3,500 *less* calories to lose that damn pound. So, if you reduce your caloric intake by 500 calories per day for one week you will lose one pound. Over a year this could add up. And, of course, the converse is true.

- Sitting burns about 30 to 50 calories an hour for children, while running around outside and playing for an hour burns 400 to 500 calories, depending on the weight of the child. Sitting burns 80 calories in the adult per hour—get up and mow the lawn and you'll burn 325 calories per hour. Better yet, take your "schweethaht" dancing and burn 395 calories per hour. If sports are your "schtick," swimming is tops at burning 790 calories per hour. Volleyball is very low on the calorie-burning pole using only 215 calories per hour. Golf burns 250 per hour if you are using a cart, kick it up to 350 per hour if you are walking and swinging a million times per hole. Head over to the gym, sign up for aerobics, actually *take the class* and burn 505 calories during a one hour high-impact workout. Go next door to the racquetball court and burn another 505 calories swinging furiously at that little blue ball for an hour. Martial arts, bicycling, and running a 10-minute mile all burn 720 calories in an hour's worth of time. So, you obviously have lots of choices to expend those extra calories and shed those unsightly pounds.

- In 1955, an order of McDonald's fries was 2.3 ounces and 200 calories; the new 7-ounce super size has *610* calories. But heck, it only costs 39 cents more—such a deal.

- Add a QP w/C (quarter pounder with cheese) to those super size fries and you have an additional 530 calories. Don't forget the super size soft drink and you have packed away 1,550 calories for *only* one meal of the day.

- Six of the nation's most prestigious hospitals have a Burger King, McDonald's, or other fast food restaurant in their hospital lobby or on the hospital property. Duke University (one of the weight-loss centers of the world) and Johns Hopkins Hospital are two of these prestigious hospitals—heck, you can visit your cardiologist and have a QP w/C on your way out. How very ironic but totally convenient.

- In 1955 Coca-Cola only came in a 6.5-ounce bottle. Today you can get your fix with a 20-ounce size. The 1955 Snickers candy bar was 1.1 ounce; today The Big One is 3.7 ounces. Only in America.

- Foods that are adding the most calories to the American diet are hamburgers, where portion sizes have grown by 97 calories. Chips and other salty snacks have increased caloric load by 93 calories, and regular sodas by 49 calories. (*THE WEEK* February 7, 2003)

- More than 11,000 new food products were introduced to the market in 1998. Of those new food products, 66 percent were candy, snacks, baked goods, soft drinks, and ice creams.

- It would take a 130-pound person two hours and one minute to walk off the calories in a McDonald's Big Mac and three hours and twenty-six minutes to briskly walk off the calories from a Burger King Double Whopper with cheese. Start walking and pick up the pace.

- Chewing sugarless gum can burn 11 calories more per hour as compared to keeping your jaw still during that same hour.

- You would burn 110 calories an hour if you were typing this manuscript. You might as well just sleep through that hour—you burn 80 calories an hour while sleeping. You could chomp on sugarless gum for that hour of typing and burn another 11 calories.

• The food industry spends more on advertising than any industry except the automobile industry. The money spent advertising any single new product often exceeds the total spent every year to educate the public about healthy eating. We don't have a chance. They're coming at us from all angles.

Can you gain weight by just looking at food? Well, *yes*. From personal experience, I know this to be true. But also, in a recent Yale University study, insulin levels increased dramatically in individuals exposed to the sight, smell and even the mere mention of charcoal-broiled steaks. Participant's bodies started converting glucose to fat even before they had taken their first bite. Here is an example of yet another incredible mind-body interaction. Unfortunately, this one has detrimental effects on the waistline.

Speaking of waistlines. It may come as a surprise to most Americans but our waists *should* be smaller than our hips. Yes, it's the sad truth. Apparently all of that fat that we store so easily in our abdomen is the so-called bad fat or visceral fat. There is just nothing that can be said positive about this midline mass of adipose tissue—it resists insulin and contributes to type 2 diabetes; it releases fat into the bloodstream increasing the risk of atherosclerosis throughout the arteries; it forms estrogen from adrenal gland precursors, thereby increasing circulating estrogen and increasing the risk of breast and uterine cancer and possibly colon cancer, and so on. So, in the world of weight loss and the prevention of chronic disease, losing weight around the abdomen is critical for long-term healthy lives. Thunder thighs, saddlebags, and piano bench ankles carry less than half the risk of all of the above chronic illnesses. And, naturally, exercise is the best bet for removing the visceral fat around the belly.

> *Let me put it this way. According to my girth, I should be a ninety-foot redwood.*
> —Erma Bombeck

Are there *any* sure-fired methods of getting rid of that fat around the hips and thighs? Only two that I know of…liposuction and dynamite. I'm not sure which one is safer.

Fidgeting and weight loss. Investigators at the Mayo Clinic have finally confirmed what many of us have already suspected. Those of us who constantly fidget are much less likely to gain weight by overeating as compared to those who don't fidget.

Non-obese patients in this study were placed on a 1,000-calorie diet, in addition to their weight maintenance requirements. Their total energy expenditure was measured through an elaborate technique that took into account variables such as basal metabolism rates, postprandial (after the meal) thermogenesis, and volitional exercise. After all of the variables were added, subtracted, multiplied, and divided, the remaining energy expenditure was classified as non-exercise activity thermogenesis, also known as NEAT. This is the expenditure due to fidgeting, maintenance of posture, and other activities of daily living. Two-thirds of the total energy expenditure proved to be in this category. Differences in patients in this NEAT category accounted for 10-fold differences in fat storage and directly predicted resistance to weight gain associated with overfeeding. (*Science* 1999; 283:212)

> *Q. Why are married women heavier than single women? A. Single women come home, see what's in the 'fridge and go to bed. Married women come home, see what's in the bed and go to the 'fridge.*

Are people really happy to be obese? Given the choice of being obese again or having a leg amputated, 91 percent of 47 formerly obese men and women preferred amputation. Eighty-nine percent of the men and women said they would prefer to be blind than obese. One hundred percent said they would rather be dyslexic, deaf, diabetic or have heart disease.

def'i·ni'tions

Obese comes from the Latin word *obesus*, meaning "whatever has eaten itself fat." The verb root is *obedere* meaning "to eat away." Adipose is derived from the Latin *adeps*, meaning "fat, particularly lard."

Obesity and exercise. The Cooper Institute for Aerobics Research in Dallas found that obese people who exercised regularly were less likely to die prematurely than thin people with lousy physical fitness. So, chock up another plus in the column for exercise. Even if you're not losing weight with exercise, the overall health benefits are positive.

Obesity reduces the life span. So, you might want to sign up for that gastric bypass. The newest study to be released by researchers reports that if you are carrying excess baggage at midlife, (their definition of midlife was 40 years of age), you will reduce your life expectancy by a grand total of three years. The more interesting finding is that even if you lose the weight later on the damage has been done. Well then, all of you over the age of 40 take note. If you remember your weight at 40 you might want to rethink whether or not it's worth all of those hours on the treadmill trying to melt away those excess pounds if a grand total of three years doesn't matter one way or another in terms of how long you'll be dieting on this earth. Another fat fact: If you are an obese female at age 40—weighing 20 percent or more over your ideal body weight—you can expect to lose 7.1 years of life. If you are an obese male at age 40, you can expect to lose 5.8 years. Apparently, the magnitude of this loss in longevity is the same magnitude as if you were a long-term smoker.

Obesity. Only 50 percent of our children engage in regular physical activity. One of every four boys and girls do not engage in activities involving exertion. Contrasted with a decade ago, today's typical child is five pounds fatter. Running a mile takes one full minute longer than it did a decade ago.

Brain cells come and go, but fat cells live forever.
—Anonymous

On the parental side, statistics are not much better. According to a recent national study, only 42 percent of mothers of children grades one through four exercised at all, and only 48 percent of the fathers. One in five adults is obese, and nearly half of adults are overweight. It is estimated that 12 percent of all U.S. deaths could be prevented with moderate physical activity. Approximately 60 percent of adults don't get enough physical activity to benefit their health.

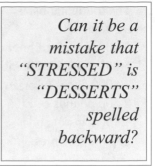

Can it be a mistake that "STRESSED" is "DESSERTS" spelled backward?

Weight Watchers. Jean Nidetch, the founder of Weight Watchers, weighed 214 pounds when she had the brainstorm to start her business in 1963. Who knows what she weighs now—she's way too wealthy to be overly concerned.

The Cardiologist's Diet: If it tastes good, spit it out.

If lack of activity were an infectious disease with these same kinds of numbers and health consequences, it would be a big deal.
—(James Hill, Nutrition physiologist, University of Colorado Health Sciences Center).

Sweet tooth. Thirty-five percent of U.S. men and women are not about to abandon all sweets for the sake of the waistline compared to 25 percent who refuse to give up meat (especially steak) and 14 percent who draw the line at giving up pizza. Only 7 percent said that they would consider giving up that good old American staple—the greasy hamburger.

French Fries and the Daytona 500. No wonder we all need to go to Weight Watchers. The following list is the type and amount of fast foods consumed at the Daytona 500:

8,000 pounds of hot dogs
5,000 pounds of hamburger
30,000 slices of pizza
2,500 pounds of French fries
7,100 cans of soda
21,900 brownies

How many calories do you expend rotating your head in a counter-clockwise direction watching those cars race incessantly around the track? Audience participation is at a minimum in this particular sport—unless you're consuming 8,000 pounds of hot dogs, 5,000 pounds of hamburger, and so on.

Gastric by-pass surgeries. We're not the only thing growing—so are the waiting lists for gastric bypass surgery, in which the stomach is reduced to the size of an egg to restrict the amount a person can eat. In 2002, 63,100 Americans had the obesity surgery, up from 23,100 in 1997. Suffice it to say that the demand for this procedure currently "outweighs" the supply.

Top 10 foods that boost sex drive according to B. Meltzer, author of _Food Swings._

1) Celery
2) Asparagus, artichoke
3) Avocado
4) Onions, tomatoes
5) Almonds
6) Pumpkin seeds, sunflower seeds
7) Romaine lettuce
8) Whole grain bread
9) Fruits and nuts
10) Chilies/herbs and spices
    (mustard, fennel, saffron,
    vanilla)

Chow down.

© Ashley Long

Junk food. Americans eat 50 percent more junk food than they did 20 years ago, including 45 bags of potato chips a year per person, 120 bags of French fries, and 190 candy bars. (*The Week*, May 24, 2002)

If you're going to eat junk food, *Why Not Eat Insects?* This is the title of a book written in 1885 and it contains recipes for such culinary delights as slug soup, braised beef with caterpillars, boiled neck of mutton with a healthy portion of wireworm sauce, and gooseberry cream with sawflies.

Comfort food. Can't get enough of that comfort food? Apparently you're not the only one. According to information collected from Information Resources, Inc, (IRI), a company that monitors spending at more than

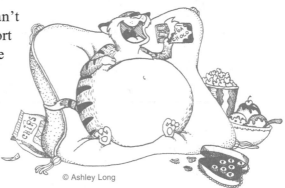
© Ashley Long

30,000 grocery stores throughout the U.S., the sales of comfort foods have skyrocketed in response to the terrorist attacks of September 11, 2001 and the anthrax scare of 2001.

In the month after the terrorist attacks, sales of frozen appetizers such as frozen pizza puffs, egg rolls, and other bite-sized morsels were up 35 percent from the same time in the previous year. The sale of Oreo cookies jumped 18 percent. Instant mashed potatoes and Cheerio sales were up 11 percent, frozen pizza sales up 8percent, macaroni and cheese up 7 percent and peanut butter up 6percent. Ice cream sales rose by 8 percent and pastries, doughnuts, potato chips and tortilla chips were all up by 4 percent.

Of course the bottom line to the increase in comfort foods is an increase in the bottom size. Packing on the calories in the form of salts and sweets relieves tension and, as an unwanted side effect, sends the scale soaring to heights previously thought unreachable.

A 29-year Big Mac attack. From April 1972 to May 2001, Donald Gorske of Fond du Lac, Wisconsin snarfed down two Big Mac's every

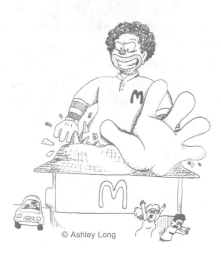

day. After finishing his 18,000th Big Mac he was assured of his spot in the *Guinness Book of World Records*. The 6-foot, 178-lb prison guard has eaten the equivalent of: 800 heads of lettuce, 820 onions, 1,900 whole pickles, 563 pounds of cheese, almost 100 gallons of special sauce, 14.5 head of beef cattle, 6,250,000 sesame seeds and 18,000 buns.

© Ashley Long

Most hazardous foods spilled while driving (from worst to not-so-bad).

- Coffee
- Hot soup
- Tacos
- Chili-covered foods
- Juicy hamburgers
- Barbecue
- Fried chicken
- Jelly- and cream-filled doughnuts
- Soft drinks
- Chocolate

© Ashley Long

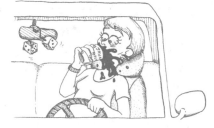

Whoa…why would chocolate be hazardous to your driving self? Think about it for a millisecond. You have just dropped a chunk of a Hershey's chocolate bar. As you try to pick it up it smears all over everything that you touch—including your freshly starched shirt and those fabulous silk pants you just purchased with your last three paychecks. You are so busy trying to remove the chunk of chocolate that your attention is on everything *but* the road. Thus it has made the top 10 list as one of the most dangerous foods consumed while behind the wheel. (*National Highway Traffic Safety Administration and the Network of Employers for Traffic Safety*—2002)

Try jogging backwards to burn more calories. Now that you have gained 10 pounds just looking at food, try jogging backwards on the way home. Jogging backward burns 32 percent more calories than jogging forward. The feet touch the ground for shorter periods of time while jogging backward, so leg muscles must work harder and move faster. If you are a runner, try jogging backward for 5-minute intervals during the normal workout.

Can eating vegetables reduce the crime rate? A report in the London *Times* provides some interesting data concerning improved nutrition and crime. British researchers found that improving the diet of juvenile prisoners reduced the number of violent offenses by 40 percent. Researchers from the University of Surrey studied 230 inmates between 18 and 21 years of age. Half of the inmates received nutritional supplements and of course, the other half received placebos. The supplements provided the vitamins, minerals, and fatty acids found in a healthy diet and the placebo provided zippo. The total number of crimes by the inmates in the supplement group was reduced by 25 percent. This study is the first to suggest that improved nutrition might be a "cheap and effective way" to reduce crime. So simple, yet it makes perfectly good sense. Now, how to implement? (Gesch CB, et al. Influence of Supplementary Vitamins, Minerals, and Essential Fatty Acids on the Antisocial Behavior of Young Adult Prisoners: A Randomized, Placebo-Controlled Trial, *Br J of Psych* (July 2002): 181 (7), 22-28)

Footnote: This may be an especially important study since the FBI has reported that the U.S. murder rate rose last year in the U.S. by 3 percent, ending a decade-long drop. There were also more robberies, burglaries, and car thefts.

Eyeballs and refined starches. Can eating too many refined starches such as white bread, white rice, and sugary cereals contribute to abnormal eyeball growth? Why has myopia (long eyeballs and shortsightedness) increased so much in the past two centuries? Why does one-third of the population in developed countries have myopia? Why is myopia

Historical Highlights

Oregon's Rajneeshee cult demonstrated that, in 1984, it is not difficult to set off a wave of food poisonings. The Rajneeshees considered a number of different viruses and bacteria, including those that cause hepatitis and typhus, but decided that for their purposes of disrupting a local election, a strain of *salmonella* would be debilitating but not fatal. At least 751 people contracted *Salmonella typhimurium* from salad bars at various restaurants in The Dalles, Oregon. The chief of the commune's germ warfare was a nurse from the Philippines, Ma Anand Puja (Diane Ivonne Onang), nicknamed "Nurse Mengele" because of her obsession with poisons, germs, and disease.

Nurse Mengele suggested poisoning the community by putting *Giardia* in the water supply. One of the members of her germ warfare committee asked her how she might accomplish this task. She replied that she would take beavers (the natural host for *Giardia)* and put them in a blender and then pour the beaver blend into the water reservoirs of the community. Was this woman a sick cookie or what? (Miller J, Broad W, Engelberg, S. *Germs* (2002)

more common in obese individuals and patients with type 2 diabetes? Could this simply be due to the diet we're eating? Researchers from Colorado State University and the University of Sydney, Australia collaborated on a study reported in the journal *Acta Ophthalmologica Scandinavia* (March/April 2002) and found that diets high in starches caused insulin levels to surge. This surge apparently affects the development of the eyeball, making it abnormally long and contributing to the development of myopia.

> *Salad eaters are at risk for parasitic disease when traveling in out-of-the-way places. My rule: watch the salad for 5 minutes and if nothing moves eat it.*
> –M. Goldberg, MD, *Diagnostic Challenges: 150 Cases to Test Your Clinical Skills*. Lippincott Williams & Wilkins, Philadelphia, 2001.

Food-borne illness. In 1990 only 13 pathogens concerned food scientists in the U.S. Today the number has multiplied 8-fold with well over 100 illnesses that are considered food-borne. It seems that nary a day goes by without some food being recalled. There are over 76 million food-borne illnesses per year, 325,000 hospitalizations due to food-borne pathogens, and over 5,000 deaths blamed on food-borne illnesses.

Some examples include:

Anasakis in raw and undercooked fish (including sushi)

Ascaris lumbricoides in imported vegetables

Campylobacter jejuni in undercooked chicken

Cryptosporidium on green onions and in chicken salad

Cyclospora on basil and raspberries

E. Coli O157:H7 in undercooked hamburgers, unpasteurized apple juice, and alfalfa sprouts

Giardia in raw sliced vegetables and fruit salad

Salmonella in raw or over-easy eggs

Salmonella in chicken

Vibrio vulnificus and vibrio parahemolyticus in oysters, clams, and mollusks (especially high-risk in individuals with low stomach acid (including the elderly population and patients on drugs that reduce stomach acid.)

Pork. The other white meat. Pork is packed with all of the essential amino acids one needs and it provides plenty of high-quality protein for a nutritious and delicious diet. Pork is a good source of the B vitamins and also provides a bit of heme iron to keep those red blood cells healthy and happy. One broiled lean pork chop has 8 g of fat (2.6 g of saturated fat), 92 mg of cholesterol, and 0.7 mg of iron.

When cooking pork make sure that it has an internal temperature of 170° F. This is hot enough to destroy all of

> **FACT:** *Infected hogs are not the only source of* Trichinella spiralis. *If you happen to be visiting the North Pole and you consume polar bear meat, you may also acquire an infection from this parasite.*

> *I had left home (like all Jewish girls) in order to eat pork and take birth control pills. When I first shared an intimate evening with my husband, I was swept away by the passion (so dormant inside myself) of a long and tortured existence. The physical cravings I had tried so hard to deny, finally and ultimately sated...But enough about the pork.*
> —Roseanne Arnold

the parasitic roundworms known as *Trichinella spiralis,* the organism that can cause trichinosis. In the U.S. less than 0.5 percent of the pigs are infected. About 10 to100 cases of trichinosis are reported to the CDC each year in the U.S. Low doses of radiation can also kill this organism, so this may be the safer pork to buy, especially in a high-risk population such as the elderly and immunocompromised.

Breakfast, lunch, and dinner. Eighteen percent of the meals consumed by Americans are eaten in automobiles. (Nationwide Insurance Company, 2002.)

Alcohol. The latest study from Harvard University Medical School analyzed 38,077 male professionals and found that those who drank at least three days a week had one-third fewer heart attacks than teetotal-

Historical Highlights

The manufacturers of Old Grand-Dad bourbon were able to produce their whiskey during Prohibition by labeling the beverage "for medicinal purposes only."

> *I'm allergic to alcohol and narcotics. I break out in handcuffs.*
> —Robert Downy, Jr.

ers—whether they had a half a drink or four drinks. Those who drank only once or twice a week had only a 16 percent lower risk. (Mukamal K. *New Engl J Med* 2003)

Alcoholism. Fifteen percent of men state that their alcoholism began between the ages of 60 and 69 years, and 14 percent report an onset between 70 and 79 years. In women, 24 percent report the beginnings of alcoholism between 60 and 69 years, and 28 percent between 70 and 79 years of age. (*Psychiatric News,* September 1998).

Historical Highlights

The shallow champagne glass was made from wax molds of the breasts of Marie Antoinette. Hardly enough to make you giddy. Wax molds of Dolly Parton's famous bazoombs might have been a better choice for the hardcore champagne drinkers.

The bubbly and the brain. The bubbles in the champagne are responsible for moving the alcohol into the bloodstream and straight to the brain faster than other types of booze. It only takes five minutes for bubbly champagne drinkers to have a blood alcohol level of .54 mg per ml. The control group, drinking flat champagne, had blood alcohol levels of only .39 mg per ml after five minutes. After forty minutes the bubbly group had blood alcohol levels of 0.7 mg per ml, just 0.1 mg short of the legal limit for driving (in England) whereas the flat champagne drinkers had only reached .58 milligrams. (University of Surrey in Guildford, U.K., 2002)

Avocados. The Aztecs were the first to name this fruit and they called it "ahuacatl," meaning "testicle." One can only guess at this reasoning but since the avocado is shaped somewhat like a scrotal sac and it hangs off of an avocado tree in pairs, one

© Ashley Long

can assume this is what the Aztecs had in mind when "ahuactl" rolled off their tongues. The Aztecs had a special recipe that they whipped up with avocados and that recipe just happens to be guacamole. P.S. If you want to speed the ripening of an avocado, place it in a paper bag with an apple.

Cruciferous vegetables. This family of vegetables has been around for somewhere in the neighborhood of 2,000 years. The name cruciferous comes from the petals that form the shape of a cross. This healthy family of vegetables contains bok choy, broccoli, Brussels sprouts, cabbage, cauliflower, collards, kale, kohlrabi, mustard greens, radishes, rutabagas, and turnips. They are considered to be the big guns when it comes to disease-fighting properties.

Broccoli comes from the Latin word *brocco*, which means "branch" or "arm." Italians brought broccoli to New York City in the 1920s and it has taken on a life of its own in this country. The average American today consumes 900 percent (this is not a typing error) more broccoli than the average American consumed in 1980. Broccoli is a potent anti-cancer agent in that its phytochemicals (phyto = plant) neutralize carcinogens. Broccoli is an excellent source of fiber, vitamin C, potassium, and folic acid. And, it only has 45 calories to boot. Sound too good to be true? Well, broccoli packs a powerful punch.

One more benefit of broccoli to add to the long list of positives. A compound in broccoli, sulforaphane, has been shown to inhibit the growth of *Helicobacter pylori*, the bacteria responsible for stomach and duodenal ulcers and the culprit in stomach cancer. This compound from broccoli was shown to kill the bacteria inside the gastric cells, where antibiotics may not be able to reach. The researchers suggested that eating broccoli along with taking antibiotics to eradicate the *H. pylori* might have a synergistic effect in patients who don't respond to antibiotics alone. (*Proceedings from the National Academy of Science,* May 28, 2002)

Vitamin C levels and orange juice containers. Betcha' didn't know this one. As soon as you open a ready-to-drink orange juice container, the vitamin C goes right out the opening. In fact, 50 percent of the vitamin C is gone after the container has been opened for seven days.

Historical Highlights

Pernicious Anemia. Dietary treatment for pernicious anemia (a type of B12 deficiency) was first introduced in the early 1900s. Patients were required to consume at least a half a pound of liver per day as their treatment for this severe, unrelenting anemia. At the time (1926), this was heralded as a lifesaving miracle; however, the actual cause of the disease had not been elucidated.

Approximately two years later, a research associate at Boston City Hospital named William Castle posed a very simple question, "Why don't normal people need one-half pound of liver per day to prevent the development of pernicious anemia?" Now William, (who flunked his course on Hematology at Harvard), knew that stomachs of patients with pernicious anemia were shriveled and atrophic, and he proposed that this may cause them to lack some very important factor that the stomach could no longer provide. How did he approach this question? His experimental protocol consisted of two consecutive periods of approximately 10 days, during which daily reticulocyte counts were drawn from the patient. (A rise in the reticulocyte count indicates that new red blood cells are being produced in the bone marrow.) During the first period the patient received 200 grams of rare hamburger steak daily, with the rationale being that hamburger meat was similar to liver in texture. During this ten-day period there was no rise in the reticulocyte count.

During the second part of the protocol, Castle himself consumed 200 grams of hamburger meat and one hour later inserted a tube through his nose to his stomach (nasogastric tube) in order to withdraw the partially digested contents of the stomach, including gastric juice. He would incubate these goodies for several hours until liquefaction of the meat occurred. He inserted the nasogastric tube down the patient from the first protocol and poured the liquefied meat from his own stomach down the tube. This is disgusting, but true. The reticulocyte count was drawn every day for ten more days and it started to rise, demonstrating that the anemia was responding to the treatment.

Castle found that neither the hamburger alone, nor the gastric contents alone, would help the patient. The combination of the two ingredients was needed in order for the treatment to be effective. He referred to the hamburger meat as the "extrinsic" factor and the gastric contents as the "intrinsic factor." And now you know the rest of the story. The extrinsic factor as we know it today is vitamin B12 and the intrinsic factor as we know it today is actually called intrinsic factor, although some still refer to it as gastric binding protein.

P.S. You may be asking yourself, "Why did the one-half pound of liver work by itself in treating the severe anemia?" Good question. Liver contains so much vitamin B12 that the mass effect of the shear amount of the vitamin was enough to overcome the lack of intrinsic factor from the atrophic stomach. Basically passive diffusion did the trick. Hamburger couldn't do it alone because hamburger doesn't have nearly the amount of B12 that liver contains.

Oxidation is responsible for destroying the vitamin C, once the container is opened. Solution: Orange juice made from the concentrate has higher levels of vitamin C to begin with. It can be used for up to 14 days after preparation and still keep the vitamin C.

Vitamin C and insomnia. Did you know that even small doses of vitamin C, taken late in the day, can interfere with sleep, especially as we age? Sources of vitamin C include citrus fruits and their juices, strawberries, honeydew, and cantaloupe melons. Other sources include dark green leafy vegetables such as spinach or mustard greens, peppers, tomatoes and tomato juice, Brussels sprouts, broccoli and cauliflower. So, when contemplating causes of insomnia in the elderly, think outside the bottle (medication and alcohol) and consider the possibility of vitamin C foods. (*American Family Physician* 2002; 65:1184)

Potomania—drinking excessive amounts of water. All you hear today is drink more water, eight to twelve glasses of water a day, increase your water intake to five to eight glasses per day, etc. Well, yes, water has numerous benefits and all of us should probably consider increasing our intake of water, *but*, let's not go overboard. Patients with potomania drink copious amounts of water for absolutely no reason whatsoever and this can wreak havoc with the kidneys and electrolyte balance. The most common "potomaniac" is the chronic beer drinker—the guy who drinks beer after beer after beer after beer. Beer is a hypotonic solution consisting almost exclusively of water. Usually when an individual consumes large amounts of beer, a state of inebriation overcomes that individual and they are too drunk to continue the consumption of the product. But chronic beer drinkers can drink without passing out. The other group at high risk for potomania is the new wave of dieters that think if they fill up on water all day and all night they won't be hungry and will lose weight. Most of these starvation diets provide less than 400 calories a day in packets of protein, salt, minerals and vitamins. So, be aware of these crash diets that require extraordinary amounts of water as part of the program. (*Lancet* 2002; 359:942)

The beauty of the cucumber. Cleopatra, Queen of the Nile, used the juice of the cucumber to maintain her beautiful skin. Her beauty secret has been passed on through the generations. Cucumber juice continues to be used today in a myriad of facial creams, lotions, and potions to maintain the health and beauty of the skin.

Cucumbers just so happen to also be used at the "other end" of the body beautiful—but for a completely different reason. The entire cucumber is consumed for this purpose. Cucumbers are the *second* most favorite vegetable for rectal consumption according to a study on the various types rectal foreign objects that have been removed from the last 20 inches of the large intestine. Of course, the question begs to be asked—what is the *number one* vegetable consumed by the rectal route? Quite a few vegetables were on the top ten list as popular items for rectal consumption.

According to the September 1986 issue of *Surgery,* carrots were number one, cucumbers were number two, bananas were number three, tied with onions (what the hell is the onion all about?) and zucchini. Some of the more interesting items that were not edible, so to speak, included sticks, broom handles, bottles, and jars. Perfume bottles were quite the rage during the '80s. Other items pulled from the depths included a cattle horn, pig's tail, ice pick (ouch, ouch, ouch), toothbrush holder, a spatula, a tin cup and a baby powder bottle. Some rectums contained multiple items. One 38-year-old male claimed a friend assaulted him and after all was said and done the following items were removed from his derriere: spectacles, a suitcase key,

> **Foreign objects.**
> *For reasons unbeknownst to clinicians, some patients have a tendency to insert all manner of foreign objects into their orifices. The children go for the orifices in the upper body— ears, nose, mouth, and trachea. Adults go for those in the lower body— vagina, anus, urethra.*
> (A Little Book of Doctor's Rules. Clifton K. Meador, M.D. 1992. Hanley & Belfus, Inc. Phila. PA)

a tobacco pouch, and a magazine. Obviously the spectacles and the magazine make sense—how can you read without your glasses? The tobacco pouch and suitcase key have me scratchin' my head. Another man inserted an entire jar of Pond's cold cream and a lemon into his rectum to relieve the pain and itching of hemorrhoids. Nary a hemorrhoid was found when the objects had to be surgically removed.

The continuing saga of fiber and its medical benefits. Is all fiber created equal? Well, for years the fiber fanatics have pushed any type of fiber—soluble fiber for healthy bowels and the prevention of colon cancer and insoluble fiber for lowering cholesterol. A couple of studies had the nerve to state that fiber wasn't a big help in preventing colon cancer, so fiber fell out of favor for this purpose. Well, the pendulum has swung back to fiber for colon cancer prevention. A group of British researchers have found a clue to why certain fiber is beneficial for colon cancer prevention. They focused on fiber that contained the simple sugar known as galactose, and found a 33 percent risk difference in the risk of developing colon cancer between the lowest and highest consumers of galactose-containing fiber. Individuals who consumed the most galactose-containing fiber had significantly lower rates of colon cancer. Fiber comes from either grain-based foods or fruits and vegetables. Galactose-containing fiber is *only* found in fruits and vegetables, and is not found in grains. The vegetables that win the gold medal for galactose are the cruciferous crew—broccoli, cabbage, Brussels sprouts, cauliflower, and kale. It all boils down to the stinky ones, once again. The more gas you have, and the stinkier it is, the better off the colon. *(Gastroenterology,* June 2002)

Lessons learned from space medicine. Fiber has been the forbidden food of space shuttles past. The prevailing theory was obvious— eating fiber would create an overabundance of fecal material with a paucity of disposal space. So the astronauts were given up to one gram of fiber per day, hardly enough to stimulate one centimeter of peristalsis, hence the major complaint of constipation in this elite group. Just as an FYI—the daily-recommended amount of fiber intake is 25-40 grams per day for all of us who are earth-bound.

Fish oil and the treatment of depression. Studies have shown that depressed patients have low levels of eicosapentaenoic acid (EPA). A British study has shown that taking 1 gram of EPA for 12 weeks can reduce depressive symptoms by 50 percent in 70 percent of the patients taking the capsules compared to 25 percent of the patients taking a placebo. (*Archives of General Psychiatry,* October 2002)

Fast food in the hospital lobby. One third of the nation's top hospitals, have on their premises at least one fast-food franchise-despite evidence linking fast food to obesity. What's up with that? Are we practicing what we preach? Obviously not. Case in point—I just happened to be teaching at a major medical center on the East Coast recently on the topic of health, food, fast foods, diet and disease, diabetes, heart disease, etc., and I happened to stroll by a Dunkin' Donuts franchise situated just across from the admitting desk in the hospital lobby. Now that's a message to convey to all of our hospital patients. Nothing like seeing the entire hospital staff queuing up to buy their cream-filled, glazed-covered, chocolate-dipped donuts.

Taking the belching out of soda pop. If you want to lose the carbonation in your soda, pour a room temperature soft drink into a glass of ice. The radical temperature change traumatizes the gas and approximately 50 percent of the carbonation will be lost. If you pour refrigerated soda into a chilled glass, you only lose about 10 percent of the carbonation. Once gas survives the initial impact of meeting the ice in the glass, it doesn't lose carbonation very quickly. Soft drinks with the most carbonation are ginger ale and lemon-lime drinks. Those with the least carbonation are the soft drinks with the fruit flavors (excluding lemon-lime). Colas and root beer fall in-between.

> *Life expectancy would grow by leaps and bounds if green vegetables smelled as good as bacon..*
> —-Doug Larson, The Albany Times Union

Historical Highlights and Candy

M & Ms were designed specifically for soldiers headed to the battlefields of Europe. The Mars Company claimed that soldiers would get a quick energy boost from a candy that would not "gum up" their trigger finger.

1894—Milton Hershey produced the first Hershey bar in Lancaster, Pennsylvania

1896—Leonard Hirschfeld unveiled the first paper wrapped candy named after his daughter "Tootsie." Based in Chicago to this day, the company makes Tootsie Rolls.

1921—Peter Paul Haligan of New Haven, Connecticut manufactured a scrumptious nickel candy bar combining the two tastes of chocolate and coconut and called it Mounds (as in Peter Paul Mounds). In 1947 he introduced almonds in the even more popular candy bar called Peter Paul Almond Joy.

1920s—Otto Shering introduced the Baby Ruth which was named after President Grover Cleveland's daughter. It was not named after the famous baseball player, Babe Ruth. Babe Ruth wanted to bring out a candy bar on his own but a court order prohibited his request.

Pepsi-Cola and "All Shook Up." Have you ever heard of Otis Blackwell? Well, he was one of the most prolific songwriters in the mid-twentieth century and he wrote the songs that will make you sing a few

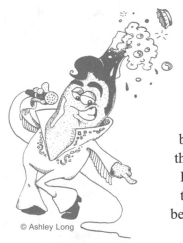

lines and start tappin' your toes as soon as I mention their names— "Great Balls of Fire" and "Don't Be Cruel" and "Return to Sender." He told his agent that he could write a song about anything. His agent just happened to be drinking a Pepsi Cola at the time and he started shaking the bottle and said, "Write a song about this." The result: "All Shook Up." Elvis Presley recorded the tune and it topped the charts in April 1957 and became the best selling single of that year.

© Ashley Long

Hunger in the womb and diabetes mellitus. Hunger in the womb may contribute to adult-onset diabetes. In research published in the April 2000 *Annals of Internal Medicine*, epidemiologists studied the years between 1948 and 1954, a period of substantial food deprivation in China. They were able to trace and test 627 adult children of women whose records were available.

They found a strong correlation between undernourished moms and children, who as adults, if their diets improved, developed insulin resistance syndrome, a condition that may lead to full-blown diabetes. It appears as if fetal adaptations to chronic under nutrition may change metabolism permanently. This can be a problem when diets improve, as indicated by the fact that the children, unlike their mothers, were not stunted as adults. The combination of the difficulty in metabolizing fat and rising caloric intake could play a significant role in the increased rates of diabetes in countries attaining prosperity.

Olives. In order to cut costs, American Airlines eliminated one olive from each salad in their first class meal service. They saved $40,000 with this cost-cutting stroke of genius.

Never mind that they are 1.6 billion dollars in debt—every little olive matters.

The onion. To the Egyptians the round shape of the onion signified eternity. The Egyptians would place their right hand on an onion when taking an oath.

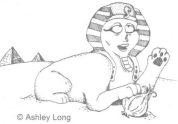
© Ashley Long

Onions. Why do raw onions bring a tear to your eye? When you slice an onion, you damage the cell walls, releasing enzymes and sulfur-containing amino acids that trigger a chemical reaction when they come into contact with each other. These volatile sulfur-containing compounds irritate your eyes and stimulate the tear glands. The irritating chemicals just so happen to be water-soluble and the flowing tears help dissolve them. When you cook chopped onions, these unstable compounds break down. Two helpful hints to reduce the tearing that accompanies raw onion cutting: Hold the onion under cold water while cutting it up and/ or chill the onion before peeling it.

Onions most likely possess these tearing compounds as a sort of chemical survival system that keeps predators away. It must have worked—onions and other members of the lily family have survived for thousands of years.

Pizza and pasta. This is basically a no brainer, but just in case there was any question in your mind, Italy leads the world in the consumption of pasta with 61.7 pounds consumed per person per year. Guessing the number two country in the world consuming pounds of pasta might be a bit more difficult. Any guesses? See Appendix A for the answer. The U.S. is number six on the list with 19.8 pounds of pasta per person.

Pizza is the word for pie in Italian. The term pizza pie is redundant. "When the moon hits your eye like a big pizza pie that's amore…" Milwaukee is the city that consumes the most "pizza pie" in the U.S.

Oysters. There's an old wives tale running around that says it's safe to eat shellfish in any month that has an *r* in it. Not true. While fresh oysters are deadliest in the summer, they can also be deadly in September, October, November, December, January, February, March, and April. The bug that causes oyster-related illness is *Vibrio vulnificus*. Eating raw oysters contaminated with this bug can be hazardous to your health at any time of the year.

According to the Doctrine of Signatures, for every part of the human body there is a corresponding object in the world of nature. For example, the testicle in the human body corresponds to the oyster in nature. The testicle and the oyster not only resemble one another, but the testicle also requires the highly concentrated amount of zinc contained in the oyster. Males with zinc deficiencies fail to produce enough testosterone and sperm resulting in erectile dysfunction and infertility.

Wine and World War II. The French helped save the Brits by an important piece of information supplied by a vintner in the south of France. The vintner informed the British that Hitler had placed a huge

> *Wine is living proof that God loves us and likes to see us happy.*
> —Benjamin Franklin (1738)

order for wine "with special corking for a hot climate." The British figured out where that hot climate was and they prepared for the Nazi invasion in Northern Africa. (Katja Thimm, *Der Spiegel*)

Wafers, Holy Communion. Often overlooked as a source of wheat gluten, the wafers given out during Holy Communion can be the source of an acute diarrhea attack in individuals with gluten hypersensitivity. Even the wafers classified as "gluten free" may still contain sufficient

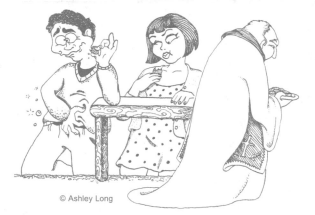
© Ashley Long

gluten to cause diarrhea. Most of the individuals sensitive to wheat gluten are classified as having celiac disease—an allergy to gluten that results in malabsorption and diarrhea.

Wake. In the 1500s lead cups were used to drink alcohol. The combination of the lead cup with the whiskey or ale would sometimes knock the person out for a few days. When found in that inebriated condition, they were often thought to be dead. They were laid out on the kitchen table and the family would gather around and eat and drink and wait to see if they would wake up, hence the custom of holding a "wake."

Chapter 8

Mnemonics for Mnemcompoops

> *The advantage of a bad memory is that one enjoys several times the same good things for the first time.*
> –Friedrich Wilhelm Nietzsche (1844-1900)

The word mnemonic comes from the Greek *mnéme,* or memory. Mnemonics is the art of improving the memory, and mnemonic devices are those that aid recollection. Students of all persuasions throughout the ages have used mnemonics to assist in remembering long lists for exam time, and medical and nursing students have been among the more clever users of mnemonic devices. This chapter is chock full of some of the more common mnemonics as well as the not-so-common ones. Perhaps a few of you will find some of these helpful for your clinical practice. (Word to the wise—a major problem with mnemonics is that one remembers the mnemonic device, but has absolutely no recollection of what it stands for).

Mnemonics for Anatomy and Physiology

Never Lower Tillie's Pants; Grandma Might Come Home. The initial letter of each word in this playful mnemonic is also the initial letter of the names of the carpal bones, conveniently listed in their proper order:

N   Navicular

L   Lunate

T   Triangular

P   Pisiform

G   Greater multangular

M   Lesser multangular

C   Capitate

H   Hamate

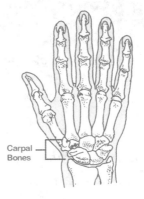

Carpal Bones

> *Baby, this party is too wild for me. As soon as I find my panties, I'm outta here.*
> –Helen Martin

* * *

The mnemonic for the twelve cranial nerves has been passed through first-year medical school anatomy class for as long as *anyone* can remember. In fact, there are two well-known mnemonics for remembering the twelve cranial nerves—the one that can be repeated at the "family values" dinner table and the "nasty mnemonic" that is usually discussed over a few too many beers after anatomy class.

The family-value friendly mnemonic for remembering the 12 cranial nerves:

On Old Olympus Towering Tops, A Finn And German Viewed Some Hops:

O   Olfactory nerve (#1)

O   Optic nerve (#2)

O   Oculomotor nerve (#3)

T   Trochlear nerve (#4)

T   Trigeminal nerve (#5)

A   Abducens nerve (#6)

F   Facial nerve (#7)

A   Acoustic nerve (#8)

G   Glossopharyngeal nerve (#9)

V   Vagus nerve (#10)

S   Spinoaccessory nerve (#11)

H   Hypoglossal nerve (#12)

The first year male medical student's beer-soaked, politically incorrect version is:
Ooooh, Ooooh, Ooooh, To Touch And Feel A Girl's Vagina, Such Heaven

* * *

The assessment of a young woman who presents with numerous vague signs and symptoms can be a daunting task. Consider the possibility of Systemic Lupus* Erythematosus (SLE) if four of the following 11 criteria are present. Use the mnemonic **SOAP BRAIN MD**:

S   Serositis

O   Oral lesions

A   Arthralgias

P   Photosensitivity

B   Blood disorders

R   Renal disorders

A   ANA titers

I   Immunologic disorders

N   Neurological disorders

M   Malar rash

D   Discoid rash

Lupus is Latin for "wolf." The use of the wolf's name in the designation of various diseases reflects differing allusions. *Lupus erythematosus* is an autoimmune disease that may present with a rash across the malar areas of the face, giving the patient a lupine or wolflike facies.

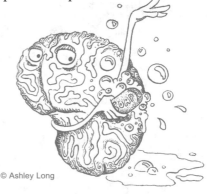

© Ashley Long

*   *   *

Rheumatic fever has a number of **fives** to remember:
    Five **major criteria**: carditis, arthritis, chorea, subcutaneous nodules, erythema marginatum
    Five **minor criteria**: prolonged PR interval, past history of rheumatic fever, arthralgia, positive laboratory tests (ESR, ASO titers), pyrexia
    Five to **fifteen** years of age primarily
    Commoner below **50°N and 50°S** latitude
    At least **five** years prophylaxis for carditis (inflammation of the heart)

* * *

Should I admit this patient with community-acquired pneumonia to the hospital? Consider the mnemonic **ADMIT NOW**:

A   Age greater than 65

D   Decreased immunity

M   Mental status changes

I   Increased A – a gradient

T   Two or more lobes

N   No home (homeless)

O   Organ system failure

W WBC greater than 30,000/mm3 or less than 4,000 mm3

* * *

Ransom's criteria determining a poor prognosis of a patient with acute pancreatitis—follow the mnemonic **Goofy LAWS**:

G   Glucose greater than 200 mg/dl

L   LDH greater than 350 u/L

A   Age greater than 55

W WBC greater than 16,000 mm3

S   SGOT (AST) greater than 250 u/L

* * *

An assessment of the newborn baby's **APGAR** score is performed at one minute and five minutes after birth:

A   Appearance

P   Pulse

G   Grimace

A   Activity

R   Respiration

* * *

The Name Game

Apgar, Virginia. Virginia Apgar was an obstetrical anesthesiologist who developed this system of scoring in 1952 to predict newborn survival. Each letter is worth a total of two points. Among full-term babies, a 5-minute APGAR score of three or less is eight times more likely to identify babies with a high mortality rate than using other well-known parameters such as measuring the acidity of the umbilical cord blood.

Mnemonic for taking a rapid history in trauma patients as they enter the Emergency Room: **AMPLE**

A   Allergies

M   Medications

P   Past Illnesses

L   Last meal

E   Events preceding the injury

* * *

Use the mnemonic **FRAIL MOM** and **DAD** for assessing the geriatric patient in the primary care setting:

F Falls

R Relative or caregiver strain

A Activities of daily living

I Incontinence

L Living situation

M Memory impairment

O Oculo-otic impairment
    (visual and auditory problems)

M Malnutrition

D Drugs

A Advance directives

D Depression

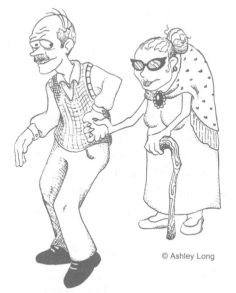

© Ashley Long

* * *

The mnemonic for the patient with an enlarged spleen is, cleverly—
SPLEEN: The following is a helpful mnemonic for the possible causes of splenomegaly (mega=big):

S   Sequestration of blood (sickle cell anemia, thalassemia, autoimmune hemolytic anemia)

P   Proliferation (increased growth) due to chronic immune stimulation (viral causes are most common)—(consider the Epstein-Barr Virus and/or cytomegalovirus)

L   Lipid-storage diseases (Tay-Sach's disease, Gaucher's disease)

E   Engorgement such as that seen with portal hypertension secondary to cirrhosis of the liver, portal vein thrombosis, or abdominal tumor compressing the portal vein

E   Endowment (congenital causes including hemangiomas, splenic cysts)

N   iN-vasion (invasive disease such as the leukemias or lymphomas; in the elderly population think of chronic lymphocytic leukemia or non-Hodgkin's lymphoma)

The ability to palpate the spleen varies with the age of the patient. The spleen is palpable in 30 percent of normal full-term newborns, in 10 percent of healthy one-year-olds, and in only 1 percent of children up to the age of 12. The spleen is non-palpable in the adolescent and adult unless it is enlarged. The normal spleen is about the size of a small fist; however, in order to palpate the spleen in the adolescent or adult, it must be three times its normal size.

* * *

The **ABCDEF**s of malignant melanoma—a guideline for the assessment of pigmented skin lesions.

How many times have you looked at a mole or change in the skin and wondered if it was a cancerous change known as the malignant melanoma or just a plain ol' mole? Since the chance of developing a melanoma is astronomical these days, it would behoove you to know some numbers and the mnemonic to assess this particular mole or change in the appearance of the skin around a mole. Let's look at some numbers, shall we? The risk of developing malignant melanoma in 1935 was 1/11,500; in 1980 the risk was 1/2,500; in 1992 the risk was 1/105; 1996, 1/87; and in 2000 the risk was 1/75. Do we see a trend here? The incidence of malignant melanoma is increasing faster than any other cancer in the U.S. Most likely this is due to our obsession with tanned skin. Now that you know the numbers, what should you consider when looking at a mole? Here's the mnemonic using the ABCs:

A   Asymmetry (one half is unlike the other; the lesion cannot be folded evenly onto self)

     Appearance of a new pigmented lesion (especially in patients older than 40)

B   Border (irregular, notched, hazy, cauliflower-like, poorly defined)

     Bleeding of the mole (or other surface changes such as crusting, erosion, oozing, scaliness or ulceration)

C   Color (irregular pigmentation pattern, shades of brown, black, gray, red or white may be present)

     Change in the shape, size, or color of the mole

     Concern of the patient regarding a skin lesion

D   Diameter exceeding 6 mm in any direction or larger than the size of a pencil eraser (in combination with at least one of the other warning signs)

E   Elevation (change in height from flat or nonpalpable), Enlargement, and Erythema

F   Feeling (presence of sensation such as itching, tenderness or pain)

(Source: *ADVANCE* for Nurse Practitioners, May 2000) (www.advancefornNP.com)

* * *

What is that SPF rating that you see on suntan lotions and potions?
First of all, figure out the amount of time that it normally takes you to develop a sunburn. For example: If it normally takes you 10 minutes to burn at the beach without any protection from the sun, an SPF-15 lotion will let you vegetate on the beach towel for 15 times that 10 minutes or 150 minutes (2.5 hours.) After that, you should pack it up and head indoors. If you stay in the sun any longer, even if you reapply sunscreen, you will burn. (A turkey will burn in the oven if you cook it too long—no matter how many times you baste it...get the drift?)

SLIP, SLOP and SLAP!! Slip on a shirt, Slop on lots of sunscreen with an SPF (sun protective factor) of 15 or higher (light-skinned folks should opt for the SPF-30 products) or new products that contain Parsol 1789 (Ombrelle, PreSun Ultra or Shade UVA Guard), and Slap on a hat. Of course, you know that you should apply sunscreen approximately 15 to 30 minutes before heading out into the sun, but for maximum protection, reapply it after 15 to 30 minutes in the sun. And use a generous amount, not a little dab. An ounce should be enough to cover all exposed skin. Thus, a 4-ounce tube contains only four applications, and you might use that much in one day—expensive, but worth it to protect your skin.

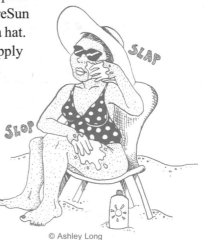

© Ashley Long

Some additional notes on melanoma:

The percentage of patients under age 30 who regularly use tanning beds may have nearly an eight times greater risk of melanoma than those who never use tanning beds.

Patients who work indoors and get short, intense sun exposure during activities such as skiing, golf, and sailing seem to have a higher incidence of melanomas. Thus, it appears that acute, intermittent exposure does the damage.

Eighty percent of one's lifetime exposure takes place prior to the age of 20. Only 9 percent of U.S. teenagers wear sunscreen. Adolescents typically have moles (also referred to as nevi) with irregular borders, multiple shades of pigment or both. Most are normal variations of the benign nevi, but any lesion that arouses clinical suspicion or is of concern to the patient should be removed by surgical excision.

A significant risk of nonfamilial melanoma occurs if an individual has more than 120 small benign moles less than 5 mm in diameter or more than five large moles greater than 5 to 10 mm in diameter), at least one mole that appears atypical (at least two of the aforementioned characteristics in the ABCD mnemonic), or a mole on the buttocks.

Malignant melanomas occur in an abnormally high percentage (about 1 percent) of PUVA-treated psoriasis victims, but the melanomas usually don't show up until about 15 years after the initiation of PUVA treatment.

Sun protection: Add a little Rit-Sun Guard® to the washing machine water to help prevent UV rays from reaching the skin. Studies show that washing your basic T-shirt in this new product increases the sun protection rating from a UPF (Ultraviolet Protection Factor) of 5 to a factor of 30. The active ingredient, Tinosorb, lasts through at least 20 additional washings.

* * *

Kussmaul respirations are defined as having a regular rhythm, however breathing is deeper than normal. The rate may be slow, normal, or fast. Kussmaul respirations are the body's response to acidosis. The patient is compensating for excess hydrogen ions by blowing off excess carbon dioxide and water. Use the mnemonic **KUSMAL** to remember the major causes of acidosis:

K Ketosis (consider type 1 diabetic ketoacidosis or a patient in the induction stages of the Atkin's diet, or a starving patient)

U Uremia (as seen in the patient with acute or chronic renal failure; the kidneys are unable to secrete the excess hydrogen ions)

S Salicylate overdose

M Morphine or other opiate

A Alcohol toxicity

L Lactic acidosis

* * *

The mnemonic **PANDAS** is used to describe a syndrome that some children develop after having a streptococcal infection. The children develop motor or vocal tics, obsessions, compulsions, or combinations of these symptoms shortly after experiencing a strep throat, specifically group A beta hemolytic strep.

P Pediatric

A Autoimmune

N Neuropsychiatric

D Disorders

A Associated

S Streptococcal infections

Historical Highlights

The clinical study of movement disorders or involuntary movements began in the Middle Ages with the descriptions of the "dancing mania." These abnormal movements had often been associated with infectious epidemics or had occurred as a component of group hysteria. The great English physician, Dr. Thomas Sydenham in 1686, described the first "dancing mania" and described it as St. Vitus Dance or chorea minor.

* * *

> *Former President Reagan seems a bit confused by all the recent furor. He called a news conference to deny ever having slept with Nancy.*
> –David Letterman

To remember the clinical hallmarks of Alzheimer's disease consider the **4 A**s:

Amnesia is defined as the loss of memory initially for recent events and ultimately for remote events.

Questions to ask family members about patients with memory problems include:

- Can you give some examples of times when the patient had trouble with memory?

- Does he or she have difficulty remembering recent events only, or is recalling things from more than 10 years ago also a problem?

- Does he or she have trouble remembering names or faces of familiar people?

- Has he or she gotten lost while driving or walking in familiar areas?

- How many times a day would you say he or she is having trouble with memory?

Agnosia is defined as the total or partial loss of the perceptive faculty by which persons and things are recognized. For example, a person may not associate a key with its purpose or may be unable to recognize words.

Questions to ask family members to determine problems with agnosia:

- Does he or she have any difficulty recognizing familiar people or places?

- Does he or she have any difficulty recognizing familiar objects or personal items?

Apraxia is defined as the inability to carry out a motor function in the absence of any motor weakness, such as having adequate muscle strength but not being able to dress oneself.

Questions to ask family members to determine problems with apraxia:

- Does he or she have any difficulty with dressing or bathing alone?

- Any difficulty with using a brush or comb?

- Any difficulty feeding himself or herself?

Aphasia is defined as a communication disorder that may include expressive difficulties and receptive difficulties.

Questions to ask family members to determine problems with aphasia:

- Does the patient have any difficulties with finding the right word to say?

- Does the patient substitute an incorrect word, such as "chair" for "table"?

- Does the patient break off in midsentence or lose his or her train of thought?

- Does the patient stutter or repeat words over and over?

The Name Game

Alzheimer, Alois (1864-1915). Dr. Alois Alzheimer was the founder of the Munich School of neuropathology and a professor of psychiatry. His greatest contribution was the delineation of the histopathology of general paresis and of organic mental diseases due to arteriosclerosis and senility (now referred to as dementia). In 1906 he first described the pathological changes in the cerebral cortex which occurred in patients with a particular type of presenile dementia, now referred to eponymously as Alzheimer's dementia or disease. Actually the newest term is Dementia of the Alzheimer's Type or DAT.

Alzheimer's initial report discussed a 51-year-old woman who "…showed jealousy toward her husband as the first noticeable sign of the disease. Soon a rapidly increasing loss of memory could be noticed. She could not find her way around in her own apartment. She carried objects back and forth and hid them. At times she would think that someone wanted to kill her and would begin shrieking loudly...After 4.5 years of the disease, death occurred."

(Steffens DC, Morgenlander JC. Initial evaluation of suspected dementia. *Postgrad Med* 1999; 106(5): 72-83. Bolla LR, Filley CM, Palmer RM. Office diagnosis of the four major types of dementia. *Geriatrics* 2000; 55(1): 34-46. D'Esposito M, Weksler ME. Brain aging and memory: New findings help differentiate forgetfulness and dementia. *Geriatrics* 2000; 55(6): 55-62.)

A website of interest: Alzheimer's Association *http://agenet.org*

> *They tell you that you will lose your mind as you grow older. What they don't tell you is that you won't miss it.*
> —Malcolm Crowley (1898-1989)

* * *

PANIC episode

P   Palpitations

A   Abdominal distress

N   Nausea

I   Increased perspiration

C   Chest pain, chills, choking

* * *

A useful mnemonic to evaluate the patient's chief complaint. It really doesn't matter what the actual complaint happens to be and that's the beauty of this mnemonic. The patient could have a headache, chest pain, limp, or any other complaint for that matter. For example, let's use the chief complaint of headache. A clinician can gather most of the relevant information from the patient's history using the **PQRST** mnemonic.

P   Precipitate or palliate: What seems to trigger the headache? What do you do to make the headache go away?

Patient: My headache always occurs when I get my period. (Big clue—menstrual migraine. Of course this only works if the patient is female.)

Patient: My headaches only occur at 3 p.m. in the afternoon when my children come home from school. (Big clue—tension headaches.)

Patient: My headaches occur every morning when I wake up. (Clue: Early morning headaches should trigger a few thoughts—1) Is this increased intracranial pressure observed after a prolonged period in the supine position? 2) Does this patient have sleep apnea? 3) Could this be carbon monoxide poisoning—how is the patient's home ventilated?

Q   Quality or quantity: What type of pain is it? Sharp, dull, throbbing, shooting, etc.

R   Radiate: Where does the pain go? Around the forehead, on the side of the head, up the back of the head?

S   Severity: On a scale from one to ten, how would you rate your headache, with one being the least pain and ten being the most pain?

T   Temporal sequence: When did the pain start? How long does the pain last? What time of the month is it? What time of the day does the pain occur?

* * *

VINDICATES is a useful mnemonic for the differential diagnosis of a patient's chief complaint. For example, if a patient complains of a headache, consider the following causes:

V   Vascular—is this a migraine headache?

I   Infections—is this encephalitis or meningitis?

N   Neoplasm (new growth)—is this a brain tumor or some other space-occupying lesion?

D   Degenerative—is this Alzheimer's dementia or Parkinson's disease?

I   Idiopathic/iatrogenic—is this caused by something the medical profession is doing— for example, a medication?

C   Congenital—could this headache have a cause based on a congenital anomaly such as Dandy-Walker syndrome?

A   Autoimmune—is this headache due to a vasculitis such as lupus?

T   Trauma—is there a history of trauma in this patient?

E   Environmental/endocrine—could this headache be due to carbon monoxide poisoning? Or an endocrine cause such as acromegaly?

S   Social—is there a reason this patient may benefit from a headache?

* * *

The treatment of angina pectoris should include all of the elements listed in the following mnemonic, **ABCDE,** according to the guidelines developed by three major medical associations.

A   Aspirin and Antianginal therapy

B   Beta-blockers and Blood pressure medications

C   Cholesterol management and Cigarette smoking cessation

D   Diet and Diabetes management

E   Exercise and patient Education

Angina is the Latin word for "sore throat"and is derived from the Latin verb *angere,* "to choke or to throttle." The most common use of angina today is associated with chest pain of cardiac origin and is referred to as *angina pectoris*, where pectoris refers to the chest. So, *angina pectoris* literally means"'choking chest."

* * *

Chest pain and the 3 Ps

Pleuritic pain (pain exacerbated by deep breaths), pain on Palpation, and pain with changes in Position are known as the 3 Ps. When chest pain is precipitated by any of these deliberate maneuvers, the likelihood of a myocardial infarction is remote. When the chest pain is reproducible by palpation or a change in position, consider a musculoskeletal cause, such as costochondritis, as the likely choice. Pleuritic pain usually points to a pulmonary source.

If two of the 3 Ps are present, one can rule out a myocardial infarction (MI) as the cause of chest pain with relative confidence. A myocardial infarction or the pain of angina pectoris ("choking chest"), occurs in approximately 5 to 7 percent of patients whose pain is reproducible by palpation; if changing the position of a patient produces the chest pain, the probability of this chest pain being an MI drops to 2 percent; and, if the chest pain is reproducible only by taking deep breaths, the likelihood of a coronary event is only 1 percent.

* * *

The following is a useful mnemonic when taking a gynecologic history from a patient:

PASs Me the GRAvy and BisCuits

P   Parida status

A   Activity (sexual)

S   STD history (sexually transmitted diseases)

M   Menstruation history (last menstrual period, regularity)

GRA   GRAvida status

BC   Birth Control

* * *

A quick differential diagnosis for the causes of shock uses **SHOCK** as the mnemonic:

S   Sepsis

H   Hypovolemia

O   Obstruction to flow

C   Cardiac failure

K   Kooky disorders

* * *

When interpreting a chest X-ray, use the mnemonic **ABCDEFGHI**:

A   Airway (Is it midline, patent?)

B   Bones and soft tissue (fractures, lytic lesions)

C   Cardiac silhouette size

D   Diaphragm (flat or elevated hemidiaphragm)

E   Edges (borders) of the heart

F   Fields (lung fields, well-inflated, no infiltrates, effusions or nodules)

G   Gastric bubble (present, obscured or absent)

H   Hilum (nodes or masses)

I   Instrumentation (lines, tubes)

* * *

When interpreting an X-ray for an arthritic joint, use the mnemonic **ABCS**:

A   Alignment

B   Bone mineralization

C   Cartilage space

S   Soft tissue

* * *

What are the indications for dialysis? Use the mnemonic **AEIOU**:

A   Acid-base disturbances

E   Electrolyte disturbances

I   Intoxication

O   Overload of volume

U   Uremia

* * *

When evaluating the causes of restrictive lung disease consider the mnemonic **PAINT**:

P   Pleural disease (effusion, etc.)

A   Alveolar process (pneumonia)

I   Interstitial lung disease

N   Neuromuscular

T   Thoracic cage

* * *

When evaluating the causes of obstructive lung disease consider the mnemonic **LACE**:

L   Local (upper airway)

A   Asthma

C   Chronic bronchitis—bronchiectasis

E   Emphysema

* * *

What are the triggers of childhood asthma? Use the mnemonic **ASTHMA**:

A   Allergy (the house dust mite, pollens, dander [cat, dog, cockroach])

S   Sport (exercise, play)

T   Temperature (cold, wet, windy weather)

H   Heredity (familial tendency to asthma; gene locus)

M   Microbiology (viruses, mycoplasma, etc.)

A   Anxiety (stress, worries)

* * *

Here's a mnemonic to assess the *severity* of asthma in a patient—use the **6 S**s:

S   School (How much missed?)

S   Sleep (How much disturbed?)

S   Sport (How able? Opting out?)

S   Social activities (How much disruption?)

S   Symptom score card (How severe?)

S   Steroids (Drug requirements?)

*   *   *

What are the **6 I**s associated with eczema?

I   Itch (antihistamines, etc.)

I   Ichthyosis (emollients, etc.)

I   Inflammation (topical steroids)

I   Infection (antibiotics)

I   Irritability

I   self-Image (psychological support)

*   *   *

Why are circumcisions performed? Use the **6 M**s:

M   Moses (Jewish religion)

M   Mohammed (Muslims)

M   Mother wants it

M   Money

M   Mythical reasons

M   Medical reasons (phimosis, paraphimosis)

*   *   *

INFECTIOUS DISEASE MNEMONICS

What are the clinical syndromes caused by *Strep pyogenes?*

PY PharYngitis

O   Otitis media

G   Glomerulonephritis

E   Erysipelas

N   Necrotizing fascitis, myonecrosis

E   cElluitis

S   Shock, Toxic Shock Syndrome (TSS)

* * *

What are the bugs that cause urinary tract infections? **SEEK Pee Pee**:

S   Serratia marcescens

E   *E. coli*

E   Enterobacter cloacae

K   Klebsiela pneumonia

P   Proteus mirabilis

P   Pseudomonas aeruginosa

* * *

What are the bugs that cause food poisoning that makes you vomit? **Vomit Big Smelly Chunks**:

V   Vibrio parahaemolyticus and vulnificus

B   Bacillus cereus

S   Staph aureus

C   Clostridium perfringins

* * *

What are the bugs that cause diarrhea? **Very Runny Caca Gets Expelled**:

V   Vibrio Cholera

R   Rotavirus

C   Cryptosporidium

G   Giardia

E   ETEC

* * *

The following syndromes/infections that occur *in utero*—this blood test is referred to as **TORCH** titers:

T   Toxoplasmosis

O   Other: *treponema pallidum* (syphilis), *Listeria monocytogenes*, *Mycobacterium* TB, Varicella

R   Rubella

C   CMV (Cytomegalovirus)

H   Herpes, HIV

* * *

INTERPRETATION OF LAB TESTS MNEMONICS

The **ABCs** of hematuria (the possible causes of blood in the urine):

A   Anatomy (cysts, etc)

B   Bladder (cystitis)

C   Cancer (Wilm's tumor)

D   Drug related (cyclophosphamide, also known as Cytoxan)

E   Exercise induced

F   Factitious (Munchausen Sydrome see end of chapter)

G   Glomerulonephritis

H   Hematology (bleeding disorder, sickle cell)

I   Infection (urinary tract infection)

J   inJury (trauma)

K   Kidney stones (hypercalciuria—excess calcium in the urine)

(Clinical note: the four major causes of hematuria in children are as follows: infection, inflammation, injury, and kidney stones)

* * *

A mnemonic for the possible causes of an elevated ALT or AST (liver enzyme) value in asymptomatic patients—**ABCDEFGHI–M**:

A   Autoimmune hepatitis

B   Hepatitis B

C   Hepatitis C

D   Drugs or toxins

E   Ethanol

F   Fatty liver

G   Growths (i.e. benign or malignant tumors as well as other masses or space-occupying lesions)

H   Hemodynamic disorder (congestive heart failure)

I   Iron (hemochromatosis), copper (Wilson's disease), or alpha-1 antitrypsin deficiency

M   Muscle injury

* * *

SAD (Seasonal Affective Disorder):

As the days get shorter in the fall and winter, the faces get longer and the lower lip seems to protrude more than usual. The reduced amount of sunlight has a direct effect on the hypothalamic influence governing the production of melatonin and serotonin. Darker days mean increased melatonin, and increased need for sleep. Darker days also mean less serotonin and a decreased desire to put a smile on your face and a zip in your doo-dah. These are the classic symptoms of seasonal affective disorder (SAD)

"Darker" appears to be the operative word here; therefore "lighter" may make a difference in mood and sleep patterns. Indeed, "lighter" does make a difference. Three controlled trials, reported in the October 1998 issue of the *Archives of General Psychiatry* used bright lights for approximately 30 to 45 minutes in the morning. The bright light therapy significantly alleviated the symptoms of winter depression or seasonal affective disorder. The newer full spectrum UV light systems cost approximately $200 and are well worth the bucks if you're in the doldrums as soon as December 21 rolls around. This is the official date for the arrival of winter and has the distinction of having the least amount of daylight all year. Miami has approximately 10.5 hours of daylight on this date, Seattle has 8.5 hours of daylight on December 21, and Anchorage Alaska has fewer than 5.5 hours of daylight.

The following mnemonic can be used to evaluate a patient with suspected depression—there is a short mnemonic, SALSA that works beautifully in primary care settings and a longer mnemonic that fits the world of psychiatric evaluation:

S   Sleep disturbances (either too much or too little—hypersomnia or insomnia)

A   Appetite changes (either too much or too little)

LS Low Self-esteem

A   Anhedonia (the loss of interest in day-to-day activities)

* * *

The longer mnemonic for major depression is used by psychiatric professionals. The patient must exhibit five of the following symptoms during the same two-week period and these symptoms must represent a change from the previous functional status. At least one of the first two symptoms listed must be included in the five:

SIG: E Caps (Prescribe energy capsules):

S   Sleep (insomnia or hypersomnia)

I   Interest (loss of interest or loss of pleasure in activities)

G   Guilt (feeling of excessive guilt, worthlessness, hopelessness)

E   Energy (fatigue or loss of energy)

C   Concentration (diminished ability to concentrate, indecisiveness)

A   Appetite (decreased or increased appetite, weight loss or gain of more than 5 percent of body weight)

P   Psychomotor retardation or agitation

S   Suicidality (suicidal thoughts or ideation, plan or attempt, includes thoughts of death or preoccupation with death)

* * *

CRISIS—Have patients use the following mnemonic when dealing with serious illness:

C   Cry

R   Read and gather information

I   Identify your personal and family needs

S   Seek support

I   Involve yourself in treatment decisions

S   Spend time searching your heart

(Edwina Perkins, Patient; Dr. William Larimore, Kissimmee, Florida)

* * *

With the aging population today, dementia is becoming a major diagnostic challenge. Use the following mnemonic to consider the causes of *non*-Alzheimer's **DEMENTIA**:

D Drugs (especially drugs with anticholinergic properties)

E Emotional disorders (Is this dementia, depression, or delirium?)

M Metabolic disorders (consider thyroid dysfunction)

E Eye or ear disorders (check the patient's hearing and vision)

N Nutritional deficiencies (B12 deficiency tops the list)

T Tumors or trauma (malignant or benign tumors, space-occupying lesions such as a subdural hematoma, trauma such as dementia pugilistica or punch drunk—think boxing—think Muhammed Ali)

I Infections (Is this AIDS dementia or some other form of encephalitis, eg, West Nile virus or other viral causes of encephalitis?)

A Atherosclerosis complications (hypertension, carotid stenosis)

* * *

The **6 Fs** for the patient with a distended abdomen:

F Fluid (Could this patient have liver disease, heart failure or kidney failure?)

F Feces (Does this patient have a stool impaction?)

F Flatus (Excessive gas may be a cause of abdominal distention)

F Fetus (Is pregnancy a possibility? Remember that 50 percent of the women in the U.S. are surprised by the diagnosis of pregnancy!)

F Fat (Could this just be an extra bit of adipose tissue?)

F Fibroid (or other tumor)

* * *

The **6 Fs** for a woman with gallbladder disease:

F   Fair (light hair, light skin)

F   Fat (self-explanatory)

F   Forty (and over)

F   Fertile (lots of kids)

F   Female (self-explanatory)

F   Flatulant (lots of gas)

* * *

The mnemonic for an older individual with urinary incontinence (loss of bladder control) is **DIAPPERS**:

D   Delirium

I   Infection

A   Atrophic vaginitis or urethritis

P   Pharmaceutical causes

P   Psychological causes

E   Endocrine causes

R   Restricted mobility

S   Stool impactions/Smoking

* * *

Reversible causes of urinary incontinence can be determined by using the mnemonic **DRIP**:

D   Delirium

R   Restricted mobility
     Retention (urinary)

I   Infection
     Inflammation
     Impaction (fecal)

P   Pharmaceuticals
     Polyuric states

* * *

How about the **4 Ds** for the signs and symptoms of brainstem dysfunction?

D Diplopia (double vision)

D Dysphagia (difficulty swallowing)

D Dysarthria (difficulty forming words)

D Dysequilibrium (difficulty maintaining balance)

Remember the brainstem consists of the structures from which the cranial nerves arise (midbrain, pons, and medulla) and the cerebellum. The first two Ds are signs of cranial nerve dysfunction and the last two Ds are signs of cerebellar dysfunction.

* * *

In the evaluation of generalized pruritis (itching), the mnemonic **ITCHING DX** is a useful guide to differential diagnosis. (*Postgrad Med* 2000; 107(2):45)

I Idiopathic disease

T Thyroid or other endocrine diseases

C Cancer

H Hepatic disease, HIV, hematologic conditions (malignancy, anemia)

I Infestations (eg, scabies)

N Neurotic disorder (psychogenic disorder)

G Gestational disorder (pruritis of pregnancy)

D Drug reactions

X eXcretory organ (eg, kidney disease)

* * *

RULE #267

As soon as you are gloved and gowned, the itching will begin.

—Clifton Meador, M.D.

A mnemonic for the causes of erythema NODOSUM. What is erythema nodosum? Erythema nodosum is the medical term for tender, red, ill-defined nodules under the skin that appear most often on the shins but may occur on the face, neck, trunk, or arms. These lesions are usually symmetric, gradually regress into lesions similar to bruises, and usually disappear within three to six weeks with no ulceration or scarring. (Brodell RT, Mehrabi MS, *Postgrad Med* 2000; 108(6):148)

NO cause is found in 60 percent of the cases

D Drugs (iodide, bromides, sulfonamides)

O Oral contraceptives

S Sarcoidosis or Löfgren's syndrome

U Ulcerative colitis, Crohn's disease, Behçet's syndrome

M Microbiology: any chronic infection (bacterial, viral, yersinia, tuberculosis, leprosy, deep fungal)

* * *

What are the causes of macrocytic anemia (red blood cells are too big)? A DASH of salt on the Big Mac (Macrocytic Anemia):

D Defective DNA synthesis

A Accelerated erythropoiesis

S Surface area increase (HOP – Hepatic disease, Obstructive jaundice, Postsplenectomy)

H Hoo knows—myxedema, ETOH (alcohol)

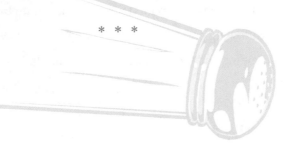

* * *

What are the causes of microcytic anemia (red blood cells that are too small)? The **FLAT MicrobeS**:

F   Fe deficiency (iron deficiency)

L   Lead poisoning

A   Anemia of chronic disease

T   Thalassemia

S   **sd**Sideroblastic anemia

* * *

Use the mnemonic **WEIGHT LOSS** to determine the causes of a protein-calorie deficit in the elderly.

W   Wandering and forgetting to eat due to dementia

E   Emotional problems (eg, depression)

I   Impecunity (insufficient funds for food)

G   Gut problems

H   Hyperthyroidism or other endocrine dysfunction

T   Tremor or other neurological problems interfering with the ability to feed oneself

L   Low-salt, low-cholesterol or other unappetizing diet

O   Oral problems (eg, poor dental care or mouth hygiene)

S   Swallowing problems

S   Shopping and food-preparation difficulties

* * *

Baron Karl Friedrich Heironymus Von Munchhausen

Von Munchhausen*, Baron Karl Friedrich Heironymus, was an eighteenth century German mercenary in service to the Russian army. After retiring from the military, he amused his friends by telling outrageous stories about his prowess as a soldier and athlete. He described his adventures in a way that bore little semblance to reality and was compelled to tell the most incredible lies about his adventures. He became well known, liked and even revered for his story telling, which lifted his spirits and increased his self-esteem. He also became psychologically addicted to the "fixes" he received from such admiration and had to continually repeat the experience and increase the bizarreness factor each time.

His fame was facilitated by a popular book and the 1989 movie *The Adventures of Baron Munchausen.* The Baron's main legacy, however, is not the fanciful musings of an eccentric storyteller. Rather, his name has become eponymous with a bizarre medical-psychological disorder. Munchausen syndrome was so named by Dr. Richard Asher (*Lancet* 1:339, 1951) an exceptionally perceptive and articulate English physician, to describe the startling and often bizarre presentation by arch malingerers who feign catastrophic illness.
*The English-speaking world changed the spelling of his name to Munchausen.

DESCRIPTION: Munchausen syndrome patients actually fake their illnesses by describing or creating unusual and perplexing patterns of symptoms. For example, they may take massive quantities of unrelated medications; they may inject themselves with urine or feces; they may deposit blood or feces in samples of their own urine submitted for laboratory tests.

An extreme case involved a young woman whose disorder began at age 16 and over the next 12 years she was admitted to 385 hospitals and received 38 operations. When she eventually had a genuine medical problem the suspicious medical community ignored her pleas for treatment. Classic Munchausen patients typically undergo a number of painful, and even dangerous,

(Continued next page)

medical procedures and treatments. Clearly this disorder is primarily a psychiatric problem associated with severe emotional difficulties. The patients are usually intelligent and resourceful and are sophisticated regarding medical practices. Their overwhelming quest for attention and motivation for forging illness appears to be associated with identity problems, inadequate impulse control, and unstable interpersonal relationships. Commonly, there is an early history of emotional and physical abuse.

Approximately 12,000 Americans have Munchausen syndrome and the cost to taxpayers is well over $40 million per year.

Beyond the bizarre Munchausen syndrome is an even more incomprehensible disorder known as *Munchausen syndrome by proxy (MSP)*. The condition is always linked to the crucial factor that a parent or caregiver, usually the mother, fabricates an illness in a child and misleads a physician into believing that the child has an illness, which needs investigation. Basically the child is used as the surrogate patient. The parent (97 percent mothers) seeks medical care for the child and always appears to be deeply concerned and protective. The child is usually under the age of six and the husband is often non-existent or emotionally distant. The mother usually has some form of medical background. Most of these mothers have failed in their careers in medicine, for example a mother flunking out of nursing school or a medical technologist being fired for emotional instability. These mothers appear to be determined to defeat the system that defeated them.

Often the stories escalate so that even more serious medical investigations are undertaken which include invasive procedures, even surgery, multiple X-ray procedures, lab tests, etc. "Doctor shopping" is also a frequent occurrence in these cases. The average time between a child's entry into the medical system and the discovery of the true cause—if that discovery is made at all, is fifteen months. The tragic outcome for children of this syndrome can be life threatening and indeed become fatal. The mortality rate is 9 percent.

Chapter 9

Funny Pharm

> *Never under any circumstances take a sleeping pill and a laxative on the same night.*
> —Anonymous

Arsenic has been used as a medicine for hundreds of years. It was discovered to be effective against syphilis in 1909 by Dr. Paul Ehrlich. Of course, an overdose of arsenic is a problem and has been used intentionally in many potions and lotions to hasten death in unsuspecting individuals. Arsenic has been found in many of the herbal products that come from mainland China to the United States. You may want to be aware of this fact when purchasing herbal therapies from China since a slow deterioration from subclinical arsenic poisoning can be more of a risk than a benefit from these herbal products.

Napoleon's final days were spent suffering from diarrhea, nausea, vomiting, lethargy, muscle weakness, and a feeling of pins and needles. The pins and needles are known as paresthesias in the world of neurology. Apparently Napoleon was being slowly poisoned with arsenic during his last days, however, the source of the arsenic remains a mystery. One possibility was Fowler's solution, a therapeutic tonic that contained sodium arsenite. Another possibility would be foul play.

A prescription for arsenic. A woman walks into a pharmacy and asks the pharmacist for some arsenic. He asks, "What for?" She says, "I want to kill my husband." He says, "Sorry, I can't do that." She then reaches into her handbag and pulls out a photo of her husband with the pharmacist's wife and hands it to him. He looks at her and says, "You didn't tell me you had a prescription."

Aspirin. Over 70 million pounds of aspirin are produced annually throughout the world. Americans take more than 20 billion aspirin per year, making it America's most widely used drug. The range of clinical uses of aspirin is mind-boggling. Its anti-inflammatory effects and anti-platelet effects reduce the risk of ischemic (lack of oxygen to the brain as a result of a clot or thrombus) strokes and heart attacks. Aspirin reduces the formation of polyps in the colon, which in turn decreases the risk of colon cancer. Aspirin inhibits prostaglandin synthesis in the hypothalamus and lowers the temperature in febrile individuals. Low-dose aspirin plays a role in reducing the incidence of preeclampsia in pregnancy. Aspirin displaces thyroid hormone from its binding sites, increasing the circulating "free" form of thyroid hormone.

A new use for aspirin—fertility boost? The June 1999 journal of *Fertility and Sterility* reports that low doses of aspirin may help infertile women get pregnant. Women undergoing *in vitro* fertilization who took 100 mg of ASA daily along with follicle-stimulating drugs (fertility pills) produced twice as many eggs each month as those who didn't take aspirin. With all of those eggs being fired out of the ovary, they were 50 percent more likely to become pregnant.

A new route for aspirin—rectal? A personal story. Of course we all make mistakes during our training years and this just so happens to be the one that stands out in my mind as my biggest, albeit funniest mistake. At least the patient survived this encounter with my naiveté.

The story begins as I am one month away from graduating from nursing school. My assignment was to be Head Nurse for the Day, which, of course, meant that I was responsible for an entire unit of patients for an interminable 8-hour shift. I felt quite puffed up knowing I was among the best and the brightest my nursing school had to offer. In fact, I was downright cocky in my assumption that I knew just about everything there was to know about patient care. After all, I was going to graduate in a month and what else could I learn?

So, I prepared myself for all of my Head Nurse duties. And, in fact, I stayed up most of the night prior to the big day, preparing for each patient, each medication, and each clinical condition. I pored over every chart, looked up every drug interaction, knew the patients' psychosocial status, and all of their family members. In other words, I could not have been more prepared for the challenge.

After morning report was finished, I quickly began preparing all of the early morning medications for the unit. As I was completing my first daunting task the nursing assistant on my team came up to me and said there was a woman in room 208 with a temperature of 105° F. I almost panicked thinking that someone could *die* with a temperature that high, so I immediately stopped what I was doing and quickly snatched up the patient's chart. Fortunately there was an order for aspirin if her temperature was greater than 102° F. In fact, the order read, Bayer aspirin, grains 10, per rectum for a temp greater than 102° F. Well, I said to myself, this is a piece of cake.

So I went to the cabinet and grabbed a pair of gloves, some KY jelly (a lubricant), and two Bayer aspirin out of the bottle. I marched right down to her room and commanded her to roll over on her side, explaining that I was going to give her something for her elevated temperature. I pulled the gloves on, squirted the KY jelly on the index finger of my right hand, placed the aspirin on the jelly, opened up her buttocks with my left gloved hand, and shoved those aspirin straight up her rectum. She jumped a bit, rolled over, looked me right in the eye and said, "Don't they use suppositories for that kind of thing?"

I nearly choked, but maintained my composure long enough to quietly say, "Yes, they do, but the suppositories haven't come up from the pharmacy yet." I quickly turned on my heel, exited the room, and ran the 100-yard dash to the refrigerator at the nurses' station. I opened the refrigerator door and there sat a huge box of Aspirin suppositories—bigger than life. I grabbed one of the suppositories, another packet of KY jelly, two more gloves and raced back to her room. I was completely out of breath as I wheezed, "You're in luck! The aspirin suppositories have just

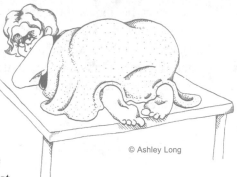

© Ashley Long

come up from the pharmacy…roll over!" She quietly complied with my command. I pulled the gloves on, removed the foil from the suppository, squirted the KY jelly on the index finger of my right hand, placed the suppository on the jelly, opened up her buttocks with my left hand and much to my surprise the two previously inserted aspirin squirted out of her rectum like two greased pigs. Bam! Bam! I shoved the suppository up her rear end, grabbed the two Bayer aspirin off the bed and fled down the hall, horrified at my own ignorance. I quietly put the Bayer aspirin back in the bottle (just kidding) and didn't tell a soul.

Later that day the nursing assistant came up to me and said, "You know that patient in room 208? She said you were the dumbest nurse she's ever had and that you shoved two Bayer aspirin right up her rear end." I sputtered a few times and came up with a brilliant line, "Well you know that a temperature of 105° F can make you delirious!" Then I admitted my mistake and pleaded with her, "Please don't tell my teacher. I'm supposed to graduate in one month!" My secret was safe with her and I graduated on time with nary a blemish on my clinical record. My teacher was treated to that story as we celebrated the graduation of my class. She roared, tears rolling down her face, and admitted that I would have graduated anyway.

Confusing drug names. Many drugs in the world of medicine have brand names and generic names that sound alike. This can be quite confusing to patients, physicians, and pharmacists and errors have been made when prescribing and dispensing these drugs. The two most confused drugs today are Celexa (an antidepressant) and Celebrex (an anti-inflammatory).

Historical Highlights and Psychotropic Drugs

The infamous Dr. Sigmund Freud was a firm believer in the healing powers of cocaine. He encouraged friends and patients to partake in this wonder drug. He told them that "the psychic effect of cocaine consists of exhilaration and lasting euphoria which does not differ from normal euphoria of a healthy person," and that "absolutely no craving for further use...appears after the first or repeated taking." Freud has since been proven wrong as we all know; however, as late as 1985 *The Comprehensive Textbook of Psychiatry* still claimed that a little bit of cocaine, "if used moderately and occasionally...creates no serious problems."

The first minor tranquilizer (the class of drugs known as the benzodiazepines) to hit the market in the 1960s was Librium. The slogan promoting this new drug was "Whatever the diagnosis...Librium." In other words, take it for anything that ails you—from bunions to brain tumors. Since the introduction of Librium, a veritable potpourri of benzodiazepines have made their way into the minds of the American public. The minor tranquilizer Valium (diazepam) became the world's most widely prescribed medication in the 1960s; by 1970 one American woman in five was taking a minor tranquilizer. This class of drugs became known as "mother's little helpers."

Timothy Leary, the famous psychologist in the early 1960s was a staunch proponent of the hallucinogenic properties of LSD. In the 1970s and 1980s psychotherapists recommended the drug Ecstasy as a means of facilitating insight-oriented therapy. It was a well-known fact that Ecstasy could not only cause permanent neurotransmitter dysfunction, but could also lead to life-threatening cardiac arrhythmias and cerebral hemorrhages—but therapists were still "high" on Ecstasy as an adjunct therapy. Ecstasy is still one of the popular nightclub drugs and it *still* causes permanent neurotransmitter dysfunction. In fact, chronic deficiencies of serotonin and dopamine have been linked to Ecstasy use. Chronic serotonin deficiency results in chronic depression and low self-esteem while dopamine deficiencies in the basal ganglia of the brain increases the risk of Parkinson's disease in these individuals.

How do drugs get their names?

Ansaid is an acronym for A Nonsteroidal Anti-Inflammatory Drug.

Asendin (amoxapine) is an antidepressant whose name suggests that spirits "ascend" or rise with its use.

Astroglide is a vaginal lubricant. "Astro" is a combining form meaning *of a star* (astral body) and you can figure out the rest— "glide me to the stars."

Atropine or Tincture of Belladonna is Italian for "beautiful lady." Ancient women would ingest the leaves of the nightshade plant (from which atropine is derived) to induce mydriasis, or dilated pupils. Dilated pupils were considered to be alluring and attractive to those of the opposite sex. Actually this is true even today. Volunteers were asked to choose between two "identical" pictures of the same person. One picture had been altered to show large, dilated pupils and the other picture had been altered to show pinpoint, constricted pupils. The volunteers were 100 percent consistent. They chose the picture with the dilated pupils every time as the "prettiest" one.

Bacitracin In 1943 a culture was taken from a contaminated wound at the site of a compound fracture of a young girl named Margaret Tracy. The culture grew an aerobic, gram-positive, spore-producing bacillus known as *Bacillus subtilis.* Bacitracin is an antibiotic produced by the Tracy I strain of *Bacillus subtilis.*

Barbiturate In 1863 a German chemist named Adolf von Baeyer (yes, the same guy that started The Bayer Company), synthesized a chemical by combining malonic acid and urease. The two substances were obtained from urine specimens from his favorite Munich waitress named Barbara—and he subsequently named the drug for her.

Calcimar (calcitonin), literally means "calcitonin from the sea." This drug is obtained from salmon, whose calcitonin is compatible with that of humans.

Dismiss (meclizine) dismisses dizziness.

Halcion was named for a mythical bird, most likely the kingfisher. This bird was believed to have the capacity to calm the wind and the sea. As an adjective, halcyon means tranquil or peaceful.

Heroin Heroin was commercially introduced to the world in 1898 as a semisynthetic derivative of morphine. The Bayer Company of Germany and Dr. Heinrich Dreser, the director of Bayer's drug research department, coined the name from the German term *heroisch*, meaning "heroic, strong." Dreser claimed that heroin had twice the potency of morphine, but that it was a safe and non-addicting drug. Kind of reminiscent of Freud's claims that cocaine was non-addicting and safe, eh? In fact, heroin was advertised as a cure for morphine addiction, just as morphine was touted, years earlier, as a cure for opium addiction. Of course, we now know that Dreser, like Freud, was absolutely clueless concerning the addictive potential of heroin.

Insulin The hormone that controls blood sugar, insulin, is produced from little clumps of cells in the pancreas. These clumps of cells, also known as "islands" are scattered through the tail end of the pancreas. The name "insulin" originated from the Latin word *insula,* meaning "island."

Lasix's (furosemide) name is derived from the duration of its effect, lasting approximately six hours.

Lobac is a muscle relaxant and pain reliever for, you guessed it, the low back.

Morphine was named for the ancient god of sleep and dreams, Morpheus. The patient feels as if he is "wrapped in the arms of Morpheus" after a dose of morphine.

Premarin (conjugated equine estrogen) is an abbreviation of three words—*pre*gnant *ma*re's u*rine*. The estrogen is extracted from the urine of a pregnant horse.

> **Luria's Law.** *Three antibiotics equal one fungal infection.* (Matz, R. *Principles of Medicine*, NY State Journal of Medicine 77; 99-101, 1977.)

Patients with arthritis have mistakenly been given Celexa, the antidepressant for their joint pain. After about six weeks the arthritic patients stated that they felt better and seemed to be happier, although their joints were still quite painful. Depressed patients have mistakenly taken Celebrex for their depression. They commented that nothing hurt, but that they still seemed to be a little down and out.

Calcium channel blockers as male contraceptive pills. When a sperm encounters an egg for the very first time it must have a special protein on its head in order to penetrate the outer protective zone. Without this binding protein the sperm cannot fertilize the egg. In order for this protein to be produced, calcium must pass through special channels in the sperm's cell membrane. Think of this special mechanism as a Black and Decker drill that needs calcium for a kick-start.

Calcium channel blockers are drugs that reduce blood pressure by blocking calcium channels in the peripheral blood vessels. Unbeknownst to researchers initially studying these drugs, the same calcium channel blockers exist on the head of the sperm. Young men taking calcium channel blockers for hypertension were reporting problems with fertility. So, the Black and Decker drill couldn't get jump-started. The sperm were knockin' at the door, but couldn't get in, so to speak. For this reason, calcium channel blockers are currently under investigation as possible male contraceptive pills. (Yeah, but would you trust him to take his pill?)

How many pills are you taking per day? A new eye-popping survey tells us that pill-popping is on the rise. Eighty percent of American adults take at least one type of medication daily—whether it is a prescription drug, an over-the-counter remedy, or an herbal potion, lotion or tincture. The most commonly used drugs appear to be the over-the-counter pain relievers—aspirin, ibuprofen, and acetaminophen. And, contrary to popular belief, these drugs can interact with everything but the kitchen sink. The most medicated population appears to be women over 65. Men between the ages of 18 and 44 are the least medicated. Well, I had better clarify that last statement. Men between the ages of 18 and 44 are the least medicated with prescription and over-the-counter drugs and the most medicated with illegal and illicit drugs. Take heed, practitioners. Ask about all drugs, big and small, legal and illegal.

Compliance and pill taking. Even though we are a pill-poppin' society, our compliance rates for prescribed medications is poor. A study utilizing computerized pill bottles has confirmed just how poorly Americans comply with taking prescription medications. The compliance rate is inversely related to the number of pills prescribed per day. For a once daily pill (e.g., oral contraceptive pill, digoxin for the heart in the a.m.) the compliance rate is 81 percent. The compliance rate falls to 77 percent with a pill that needs to be taken three times a day, and tumbles to a miserable 39 percent with a pill taken four times per day.

What are the consequences of non-compliance? It is estimated that non-compliance leads to 125,000 deaths per year, 20 million lost work days, and thousands of hospitalizations per year. One study showed that of the 93 percent of the patients who fill their initial prescriptions, only 68 percent return for the refill when ordered, and 15 percent stop taking their first prescription prematurely.

Gold dust and powdered emeralds. During the Middle Ages when the Black Death killed a third of Europe's population, university-trained physicians used concoctions of powdered emeralds and gold dust for their wealthiest patients. The prevailing theory was that the therapeutic value varied directly with the cost—the greater the cost, the better the treatment. Emeralds and gold wouldn't help even the richest patients nor would various herbal remedies, witch potions, or pockets full of posies. Since nary a treatment worked to cure the plague, the joke during medieval times was "If you want to be cured of I don't know what, take this herb of I don't know what name, apply it I don't know where, and you will be cured I don't know when." Even Leonardo Da Vinci threw his two cents in with a gentle warning to "keep clear of the physicians, for their drugs are a kind of alchemy concerning which there are no fewer books than there are medicines." Sound familiar?

Belladonna (Italian for "beautiful lady") is an extract of the leaves and roots of the plant *Atropa belladonna,* also known as the "deadly" nightshade plant, deadly being the operative word here. Belladonna exerts potent anticholinergic effects—one such effect is papillary dilation. As the story goes, tincture of belladonna was taken by Italian ladies to induce dilated pupils, a look that was considered to be quite fetching. Atropine, the name given to the principal alkaloid of belladonna, also has a feminine connection in its derivation from Atropos, one of the trio of mythological Fates. According to Greek mythology, the trio of Fates were the daughters of Themis, who served as counsel to Zeus. The three daughters spun the web of destiny for all mankind, with the daughter Atropos making the final irrefutable decision. Atropos was always shown holding a pair of shears. Presumably she used the shears to cut the threads that all human lives hang by—in other words, once Atropos approached you with her shears, the party was over. Atropine, the drug, can also kill you, as it is derived from the "deadly" nightshade plant.

Atropine poisoning. The classic picture of atropine poisoning: Hot as a hare (fever), blind as a bat (dilated pupils), dry as a bone (dry mouth and eyes), red as a beet (vasodilated), and mad as a hatter (confused and possibly hallucinating).

Atropine as a component of witch's brew ("Witche's Brew"). Three plants—*Atropa belladonna (nightshade), Hyoscyamus Niger (henbane),* and the *Mandragora officinarum (mandrake),* have a rich and vivid history as plants used for poisoning purposes, for soothsaying, for magic and for witchcraft. In ancient Greece, it was believed that inhaling a smoldering henbane plant made one prophetic. (Henbane, by the way, is the plant from which Scopolamine is made, and Scopolamine, as we know it in clinical medicine, induces "twilight" sleep.) In ancient Rome wine was mixed with the deadly nightshade plant to experience hallucinations.

The writings of the Middle Ages are replete with stories of witch-craft and devil worship. None other than Anres Laguna, the physician to Pope Julius III in 1545, wrote one such description of a "green unguent" (ointment) known as Witche's Brew: "…a jar half-filled with a certain green unguent…with which they were anointing themselves…was com-posed of herbs…which are hemlock, nightshade, henbane, and mandrake: of which unguent…I managed to obtain a good canister full…which I used to anoint from head-to-toe the wife of the hangman (as a remedy for her insomnia). On being anointed, she suddenly slept such a pro-found sleep, with her eyes open like a rabbit (she also fittingly looked like a boiled hare), that I could not imagine how to wake her…"

As the story continued in Dr. Laguna's writings, she was finally aroused 36 hours after her "anointment" with the green stuff. When she was awakened, she appeared to be quite grouchy about being disturbed from her deep sleep. She snapped at the good doctor: "Why do you wake me at such an inopportune time? I was surrounded by all of the pleasures and delights of the world." Upon further questioning, she de-scribed the pleasures and delights as vivid episodes of flying and orgas-mic adventures. She experienced evenings of debauchery at various banquets, music halls, and dances, where she "coupled with young men" with which she "desired the most."

At some point in the Middle Ages it was discovered that if the con-stituents of Witch's Brew were combined with fats or oils they would penetrate the skin and could be easily absorbed through the sweat glands in the axillary areas (armpits) or body orifices (vagina and rectum, be-ing the two that come to mind). You might ask at this point, why the oral route was not considered—the potion was too deadly if taken by mouth. Application of the ointment via the armpits or "private parts" allowed the psychoactive drugs to reach the bloodstream and brain without pass-ing through the GI tract and risking poisoning from the metabolic prod-ucts of liver metabolism.

Numerous writings from the Middle Ages contain statements about the mode of application of the "Witches salves" or "Witches ointments." For example, in the writings of Lady Alice Kyteler in 1324, the inquisi-tors states:

"...in rifling the closet of the ladie, they found a pipe of ointment, wherewith she greased a staffe (ie, broomstick), upon which she ambled and galloped through thick and thin." Whoopee! In another writing from the fifteenth century records of Jordanes de Bergamo: "... But the vulgar believe, and the witches confess, that on certain days and nights they anoint a staff and ride on it to the appointed place or anoint themselves under the arms and in other hairy places..."

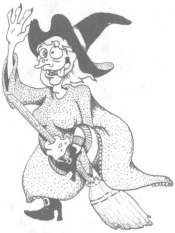

© Ashley Long

And now, you know the rest of the story. This, my faithful, readers, is why so many of the pictures during the period of the Middle Ages, depict the witches riding broomsticks through the sky! Gives new meaning to the term—riding the witch's broomstick, does it not?

Speaking of witches and potions. One of the best-known potions in the English literature came from Shakespeare's *Macbeth:*
Double, double toil and trouble;
Fire burn and cauldron bubble.
Fillet of a fenny snake,
In the cauldron boil and bake;
Eye of newt, and toe of frog,
Wool of bat, and tongue of dog,
Adder's fork, and blind-worm's sting,
Lizard's leg, and howlet's wing,
For a charm of powerful trouble,
Like a hell-broth boil and bubble.
Double, double toil and trouble,
Fire burn and cauldron bubble.
Scale of dragon, tooth of wolf,
Witches' mummy, maw and gulf
Of the ravin'd salt-sea shark,
Root of hemlock digg'd i' the dark

Liver of blaspheming Jew,
Gall of goat, and slips of yew
Sliver'd in the moon's eclipse,
Nose of Turk, and Tartar's lips,
Finger of birth-strangled babe
Ditch-deliver'd by a drab,
Make the gruel thick and slab:
Add thereto a tiger's chaudron,
For the ingredients of our cauldron.
Double, double toil and trouble;
Fire burn and cauldron bubble.
Cool it with a baboon's blood,
Then the charm is firm and good.

Whoa…take a quick gander at the ingredients listed above and be thankful for plain old aspirin. Eye of the newt? Toe of the frog? Snake's tongue? Lizard's leg? Even a finger of a dead baby was thrown in along with a piece of liver from a Jew and a bit of nose from a Turk. Now this was a poison potion if there ever was one in the annals of pharmacotherapeutics.

The treatment of tuberculosis ("consumption"). The methods of prevention and treatment of tuberculosis depended on whether you were rich or poor. Peasants preferred goat's milk or asses' milk; however, sucking on the breast of a wet nurse was even better for the prevention of consumption. Peasants also sat in a barn inhaling cow vapors as a means of preventing the dreaded consumption.

The rich, who eschewed any animals except horses, preferred travel and rest as their treatment; in fact, most of the world's great tourist routes follow the old tubercular paths winding their way to sunshine and fresh mountainous air. The most famous resorts were located on the Swiss mountaintops and they catered to the rich and famous. The Swiss drug companies prospered, the Swiss banks were full to the brim and life was good for all of those hacking and spitting from TB. Once TB was conquered, those fabulous TB resorts became Switzerland's most famous ski resorts. Do you think the linoleum has been removed from the chalets of St. Moritz by now? The British and German "consumptives" invaded the Mediterranean Riviera. American "lungers" vacationed in Albuquerque and Tucson

Does fresh air and sunshine really kill the tubercle bacillus? The answer is yes, but only the sunshine has the active ingredient. Actually, sunshine triggers the production of vitamin D in the skin and vitamin D stimulates macrophages to devour the tubercle bacillus. In addition, ultraviolet light from sunlight can kill the tubercle virus in the air.

Other treatments for TB throughout the ages have included leeching, phosphoric acid, ether, digitalis, carbolic acid inhaled for eighteen months, and boa constrictor feces. Whoa, let's back up here. How did boa constrictor feces get added into the regimen? Beats me.

As progress was made in medicine the treatment for TB progressed to removing single ribs to entire rib cages, collapsing a lung, countless X-rays and the injection of gold salts. The gold salts injections contributed to the demise of the patient by destroying the stomach and killing the liver. In other words, TB was the least of their problems after gold salts were introduced. Perhaps boa constrictor feces would have been a bit gentler on the internal organs.

Cannabinoids for pain. The use of marijuana to relieve pain dates back as far as 315 A.D. The evidence: the skeletal remains of a young girl in a tomb near Jerusalem buried with a gray carbonized material and bronze coins. The bronze coins in the tomb were dated between 315 A.D. and 392 A.D. Analysis of the carbonized material revealed the remnants of marijuana.

References to marijuana as a pain reliever are scattered throughout the annals of medical history. Studies on animals have recently demonstrated natural receptors for cannabinoids in various pain modulating areas of the brain, brain stem, and peripheral nervous system. Specific areas include the rostral ventromedial medulla (RVM)—an area in the lower brainstem that modulates pain perception, as well as the site of damage in the periphery. Cannabinoid substances produced by our own nervous system activate the RVM cells that stop pain signals and inactivate the RVM cells that trigger pain signals. In addition, cannabinoid substances block pain-enhancing molecules released after direct injury to somatic tissue and inhibit the transmission of the pain impulse to the spinal cord.

Early research shows that cannabinoids may be effective in treating peripheral neuropathy. Researchers have found that a low dose of cannabinoid offers relief of neuropathic pain in animal models. The animals, unfortunately, had the significant side effect of cognitive impairment and the other behavioral effects associated with marijuana use. (*Brain Briefings*—March 1999; The Society for Neuroscience. For more information: http://www.sfu.org/briefings)

Caught ya' lookin'. Patients have reported seeing part of their drug tablets in their stools. Yes, this can happen when you gaze into that toilet bowl after the number two and especially if the drug you are taking is called a 'sustained-release' drug. Part of the drug is released immediately when ingested; however, the part of the drug that is the "extended-release" or "sustained-release" is released from an insoluble wax matrix. So if you're looking, please note that a part of the

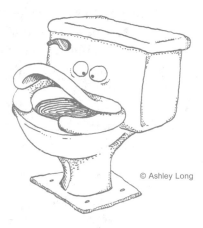

© Ashley Long

following drugs may be staring back at you from the depths of the toilet bowl: Allegra-D, Concerta, Covera-HS, Depakote ER, Ditropan SL, Glucotrol XL, OxyContin, Procardia XL, and Tegretol XL. (The XL does NOT stand for "extra large," it stands for "extended-length.")

Coffee enemas for detoxification—doin' it the old-fashioned way. Nursing textbooks from the 1920s through the 1950s touted the beneficial effects of coffee enemas for a variety of conditions ranging from arthritis to schizophrenia. The *Merck Manual* included coffee enemas as recommended therapy for detoxification until

> *King Louis XIV of France endured more than 2,000 enemas to prevent and treat disease during his 72-year reign.*

1977. Coffee enemas were dropped from the *Merck Manual* in 1977 because they had fallen out of fashion with the changing technological advances. Today, however, with the re-emergence of complementary and alternative therapies, daily coffee enemas have re-emerged as detoxifying agents in a alternative cancer therapy program known as the Gonzalez/Kelley treatment regimen for pancreatic cancer. In addition, various alternative practitioners favor coffee enemas as a means of enhancing liver function and removing metabolic toxins and waste.

The mechanism of action is presumed to be smooth muscle relaxation of the hepatic ducts resulting in increased secretion of toxins from the liver into the GI tract and out of the body. This only occurs when the caffeine is administered rectally—drinking coffee does not have the same effect on the biliary system.

Leeches. Leech is the common name for a bloodsucking worm of the class Hirudinea, but it also was, in the past (and, rarely in the present), used to designate a physician. In fact, the latter meaning came first, being derived from the Anglo-Saxon *laece,* "one who heals." "Bloodletting" or "leeching" for the purpose of treating disease caused by harmful "humors" has been utilized since before the days of Hippocrates. Since the leech was used to consume the harmful "humors" from an inflamed lesion, it was given the name "the healer." One of the most famous uses for multiple leeches was in the treatment of "dropsy," yesteryear's equivalent of today's congestive heart failure. In the 1830s bloodletting reached its peak of popularity, when 20 million leeches a year were used as bloodsuckers.

Leeches and hirudin. The drug lepirudin (Fefludan), an anticoagulant derived from leech saliva, inhibits clot-bound thrombin. (Becker RC, Merli GJ, Talbert RL. Recent strides in thrombotic therapy. *Patient Care* 2000 (August 15); 20-42)

Sweet clover and Coumadin. In the late 1920s and early 1930s, veterinarians throughout the country were warning farmers of "sweet clover disease." Cows that were eating the spoiled and moldy sweet clover were dying of hemorrhagic complications. In February, 1933, a

Wisconsin dairy farmer was distraught over the death of his favorite dairy cow from the "sweet clover disease." He decided that enough was enough, so he packed up a bale of the spoiled, moldy sweet clover, his deceased cow, and a milk pail of the cow's blood. He drove to the University of Wisconsin and demanded to know just what caused his cow's death. He persuaded a university biochemist, Dr. Karl Link, to analyze all of the items he brought with him, so he left the contents of the truck, including the bale of sweet, moldy clover, and drove home.

Six years later, and hundreds of more bales of sweet, moldy clover, Dr. Link found the link, so to speak, between the hemorrhagic deaths of the cows and the sweet clover. Link named the substance dicumarol, which is a derivative of a similar chemical known as coumarin, the substance that gives sweet clover its scent. Link also discovered the amino acid sequence of dicumarol and was able to synthetically produce it in his laboratory. The word spread throughout the veterinary world, crossed the boundaries into the medical world, and soon physicians from all over the country were beating down his door to use this substance for patients who had excessive clotting problems. Dicumarol was subsequently released as a "human" drug to inhibit excess clotting.

Link continued to experiment with the substance by producing various strengths of dicumarol. He decided that one of the more potent strengths could be used as a rat-poisoning agent. When the tasteless, odorless dicumarol was mixed with a grain, rats would devour it in large quantities and would subsequently hemorrhage to death. This rodent killer was called "warfarin," and was available nationwide by 1951.

Shortly thereafter, a young Army recruit decided that ingesting a box of rat poison would be a perfect way to commit suicide. He didn't die; however, he did hemorrhage from all orifices as well as internally. His Army doctors concluded that rat poison or "rat warfarin" was absorbed much more rapidly than "hu-

Never go to a doctor whose office plants have died.
—Erma Bombeck

man" dicumarol—as evidenced by his rapid internal and external bleeding. They began testing "rat warfarin" in humans—in small doses, of course.

Four years later, Dwight David Eisenhower, the President of the United States at the time, had a myocardial infarction while visiting Colorado. The Army physicians at Fitzimmon's Army Hospital in Denver decided to treat him with a "blood thinner," and they used small doses of rat poison (with his permission of course), instead of the human approved dicumarol. Since the "rat warfarin" treatment was successful, warfarin has since replaced Dicumarol as the oral "blood thinner" of choice.

Duct tape for warts. Applying duct tape to a wart is a less painful alternative to the common practice of briefly freezing warts (also known as cryotherapy). A recent study, published in *The Archives of Pediatrics and Adolescent Medicine* (2002 Oct; 156:71-4) found that warts disappeared for 85 percent, 22 of 26 children and young adults treated with duct tape compared with 60 percent of a similar group treated with cryotherapy. The duct tape was cut to fit over

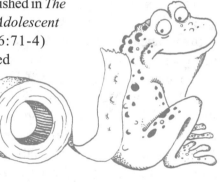

© Ashley Long

the wart and removed once a week. After removal the wart was soaked in water and then filed with an emery board or a pumice stone. New tape was applied 12 hours later. This treatment was repeated for as long as two months or until warts resolved. In the group using cryotherapy, liquid nitrogen was applied every two to three weeks for a maximum of six treatments. In both groups, most warts that resolved did so during the first month of therapy. So how does the duct tape work? Duct tape works most likely by irritating the skin thereby stimulating an immune system response that wipes out the viral infection that caused the wart.

Excuses for not taking medications.

"I think a fish ate my medication while I was at sea."

"I left my medication at my mother-in-law's house, and I don't want to go back and get it."

"I had to loan my inhaler to Elvis at K-mart."

TED vs. VED—A prescription error. An elderly gentleman presented a hastily scribbled prescription to his local pharmacist. The pharmacist quickly read the prescription made out for "TED." He proceeded to ask the patient to have a seat in the semi-private counseling area. When the pharmacist came into the waiting room and explained that he would do a "quick fitting," the patient became agitated. He did not realize that a fitting was necessary and did not want one. The pharmacist, obviously not picking up on his agitation and not listening to his protestations, proceeded to ask him if he needed "knee-length or "thigh-length." This question threw the elderly man over the edge. He vehemently explained that his urologist had not informed him that he would have to be "measured" to ensure a good fit. At that point, the pharmacist looked closely at the prescription and discovered what looked like "TED"(tight-fitting stockings for venous insufficiency) was actually "VED," for Vacuum Erection Device. The pharmacist subsequently understood the patient's reluctance to be "fitted" with other customers in the counseling area.

> *Each year, an estimated 100,000 Americans die from side effects caused by prescription medications. That's nearly 20 times the death rate caused by illegal drugs.*

Foxglove and "dropsy." The curative powers of the common plant, foxglove, were first officially recognized in 1776. The principal of Brasenose College in Oxford, England was suffering from the clinical condition known as "dropsy," a fluid overload condition in which the fluids accumulated in the most dependent parts—the ankles, legs, scrotum, and belly due to the failure of the heart to pump. We now refer to this condition of "dropsy" as chronic heart failure, or congestive heart failure (CHF). The principal attempted all of the so-called orthodox treatments prescribed by the physicians of that era, including leeching, but nothing seemed to help. He finally abandoned all of the orthodox treatments and traveled to the English countryside to the village of Shropshire. Rumor had it that a self-proclaimed witch in the village made a special potion in the form of an herbal tea for those who suffered from dropsy, so he threw caution to the wind and downed the potion. On the way out of town he started to "lose his fluid"…diuresis had set in and his clinical condition improved miraculously. Lo and behold, he recovered with such amazing speed that the news spread like wildfire. The local physicians were appalled; however, they were also smart enough to make a beeline for the village to see what ingredients were being used in the potion. Dr. William Withering was one of the first physicians to visit the

Foxglove

> ## Garlic's curative powers
> *Since Garlicke then hath powers to save from death, Bear with it though it make unsavory breath*
> —Sixteenth century textbook

little old lady and he analyzed the herbal tea and found over 20 varieties of herbs. By the way, most physicians were botanists in those days, so analyzing plants was a fairly routine undertaking. He found that the active ingredient in the potion was foxglove, the Latin name of which is *digitalis.* The name *digitalis* comes from the appearance of the plant. It has one large branch with 5 leaves at the end of it—hence, it resembles the fingers or digits. And now you know the rest of the story.

Glove compartments as medicine cabinets. The temperatures inside a glove compartment can read 50° F higher than the outside temperature. On a humid, sweltering, sleepy, dusty 100° F Delta day, the glove compartment can sizzle with temperatures as high as 150°F. Keeping medications in the glove compartment can be hazardous to your health for a couple of reasons.

The storage temperature for medications should not exceed 86°F. If you are in a pinch and medications must remain in the car for even a short period of time, put the medications on the floor and cover them with a newspaper or some other item. The floor temperature is 20°F cooler than the glove compartment and it is even cooler when something is tossed over the container.

Keeping nitroglycerin in the glove compartment can be especially hazardous to your health. Case in point—a patient with angina tossed his nitroglycerin pills into the glove compartment while running a few errands on a hot summer day. When he returned to the car the glove box door had been blown off its hinges. The nitroglycerin had heated to the point that it triggered an explosion.

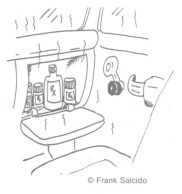

© Frank Salcido

Lithium and 7-Up. In 1929 the soft drink 7-Up was originally marketed as Bib-Label Lithiated Lemon-Lime soda. The Lithiated part was actually Lithium. It was eliminated from the formula in the mid-1940s, but it is still used as a primary treatment for bipolar disease today.

***Merck Manual* – First Edition, 1899.** The 1899 *Merck Manual* was reissued in 1999 in a centennial package with the 1999 edition. These fascinating 192 pages suggest everything from strychnine for tuberculosis to a touch of arsenic for diabetes. Arsenic was also suggested for baldness, and strychnine was prescribed for diphtheria.

Alcoholics were given opium (not a bad substitute when trying to quit, eh?). They were also encouraged to slurp up a little fresh squeezed orange juice and to drink a pint of warm water before a meal. Formaldehyde was inhaled for the common cold, sulfuric acid prescribed for nymphomania, a cigarette was suggested for asthma, and tincture of cactus was used as a blood pressure medication.

The size of the *Merck Manual* of today is a far cry from that of a century ago. The 1999 volume is a hefty 2,833 pages. However, similarities are common between the two manuals. Digitalis was the treatment for heart failure in 1899 as it is today. Quinine was the treatment for malaria in 1899 as it continues to be today. Codeine was used for the cough of 1899 and it continues to be quite therapeutic today as an antitussive (cough suppressant), even though it is not the first line therapy for today's hacking cough. So you see, some things change, some things never change. The books get heavier, the options are more numerous, but the intentions remain the same—heal thy patient (and try not to make the treatment worse than the disease).

Nitroglycerin (NTG). Nitroglycerin (NTG) has an interesting history as a use in clinical medicine. Discovered by Alfred Bernhard Nobel, this explosive material has turned into a major treatment for ischemic heart disease (angina) and, in a round-about way, for erectile dysfunction. Let's take a look at some of the more interesting aspects of NTG.

Alfred Nobel began experiments with nitroglycerin in the 1860s in his father's factory. He tried many ways to stabilize this highly volatile material. He discovered that a mix of nitroglycerin and a fine porous powder called silica was most effective. He named his product dynamite, and received a patent in 1867. Nobel endowed a 9 million dollar fund in his will. The interest on this endowment was to be used for people whose work most benefited humanity. First awarded in 1901 in his hometown of Stockholm, Sweden, the Nobel Prize is still the most honored in the world.

Nitroglycerin's vasodilating effects were first observed in the 1860s when physicians studied side effects experienced by workers in dynamite factories. The negative side effects included headaches and the positive side effects included less chest pain and heart attacks. Apparently many of these patients had coronary artery disease while working at the munitions plant; however, they had been inhaling nitrate compounds while they worked making nitroglycerin for bombs. Their arteries were in a constant state of vasodilation and the symptoms of coronary artery disease were masked. Soon after leaving the munitions plant for other jobs, their protection via the nitrate fumes was gone, and their heart problems quickly surfaced.

Have your patients ever asked you why they don't blow up when they take nitroglycerin? Well, dynamite is 75 percent nitroglycerin compared to less than 1 percent in a nitroglycerin tablet. So, unless it gets *really* hot, like it just might in the glove compartment of the car on a hot summer's day (as mentioned above), or if it's stored next to a stovetop, then it most likely will not blow up.

Nitroglycerin and a gentleman from Georgia. In 1972, a gentleman with angina from Savannah, Georgia made a landmark discovery—not only for himself, but for future generations as well. He took his nitroglycerin patch off one night (as instructed by his cardiologist) and while holding it in his hands he had an epiphany. Hmmm…. he thought. If this patch works by opening up the arteries to my heart and increasing blood flow, perhaps it will do the same if I wrap it around my penis. And, of course, without further adieu he applied the patch to his penis and "it" rose to the occasion. By increasing blood flow to his penis, our gentleman from Georgia had an erection. He was thrilled, since he hadn't seen an erection in two years. He immediately called out to his wife and said, "Mildred! Get in here!" Well, much to her surprise, there it stood, proud as a peacock. He whipped off the patch, she cuddled up, and you know the rest of the story.

Well, not quite. All she could say afterwards was—"I have the most incredible headache." The nitroglycerin was absorbed through her vaginal mucous membranes causing all of her blood vessels to dilate, including the ones in her head, resulting in a whopper of a post-coital migraine. She was not amused. He was sound asleep.

Fast forward to the present day. Medical science has since benefited *big* time from his idle patch play. Nitroglycerin has been around for years but the actual mechanism of action was not understood until recently. The nitrate in nitroglycerin boosts the release of nitric oxide from the cells lining the blood vessels (endothelial cells). Nitric oxide is the most potent vasodilator found in the body and it will open up just about any vessel.

All of this research into nitric oxide and vasodilating blood vessels culminated with Pfizer Pharmaceutical's "blue pill," introduced to the world in 1998. The drug sildenafil is affectionately known as the "Pfizer Riser" or "Vitamin V," however its brand name is Viagra. It is a potent nitric oxide booster, but specifically targets the endothelial cells of the blood vessels *below the belt.*

One important point that needs to be emphasized to *all* males reading this section and who just happen to be popping the Pfizer Riser for those special moments. If you have chest pain and you are rushed to the emergency room for treatment, one of the first questions that you will be asked as you are wheeled into the emergency room clutching your chest is, "When was your last dose of Viagra?" If you have taken Viagra within 24 hours, protocol mandates that you *cannot* receive intravenous nitroglycerin to open up your coronary (heart) vessels if you are indeed having a myocardial infarction. If the nitroglycerin and Viagra are used within 24 hours of one another, all of your vessels throughout the body can "open up" or vasodilate, and your blood pressure can fall to zero. This of course has obvious consequences—the lack of blood flow to the heart will only add to your heart attack woes, and the lack of blood flow to the brain will result in a "brain attack" or stroke. So, tell the nurse or physician in the ER *the truth* when they ask you when your last dose of Viagra was. They don't care *whom* you took the blue pill for, just whether or not you took it.

Viagra and commercial flying. A personal story. When Viagra was first released with much fanfare to the unsuspecting American population in 1998, the headlines were full of information on this new wonder drug for erectile dysfunction. As I was settling down in my seat on an airplane one afternoon to return from Greensboro to Chicago, I opened my *USA Today* and read the headline: "Pilots should not take Viagra within six hours of flying." Yikes, I said to myself, I wonder how long it's been since the pilot of this plane took his last dose. As I read further the article explained that Viagra, in high doses, could cause a "bluing" of the vision and this may interfere with reading the instrument panel in the cockpit. Geeez, I murmured. So, being a concerned passenger, I whipped out my little notepad and scribbled a note that read: "When was your last dose of Viagra? A concerned passenger in 2A." I handed the note to the flight attendant and asked her to deliver it to the pilot. All I could hear was raucous laughter from the cockpit and she came back down the aisle with note in hand. Tears were streaming down her face and she was choking back the laughter. She handed me the note. I opened it. It said: "Six hours and five minutes ago." Nobody likes a smart ass.

Generation V'ers. The year 1998 will go down in history as one of the most important years in the world of men's health. Viagra was introduced to the world for the treatment of erectile dysfunction and the Senior Sexual Revolution was "up" and runnin'. It has been five years since the introduction of that little blue bombshell and one of the interesting results of the Senior Sexual Revolution has been an increase in the rate of sexually transmitted infections in those wild and crazy 60-something's and older. The rate of sexually transmitted infections in this age bracket has increased by 300 percent since the introduction of Viagra. Woohoo!

Viagra and the tetanus vaccine. This is actually one of the 3,289 Viagra jokes that has been fired through the internet since Viagra hit the ground running in 1998: Did you hear about the woman who told her husband that she was going to accompany him to the doctor's office when he went in for his prescription for Viagra? He turned to her and said, "What are you goin' for?" She replied sweetly, "I'm gonna be getting myself a tetanus shot if you're gonna be pullin' out that rusty old thing."

Treatment of erectile dysfunction—round 2. Uprima, the second oral drug approved to treat erectile dysfunction, is a new formulation of the old drug, apomorphine. Apomorphine increases levels of dopamine in the brain. It has been used in emergency rooms to induce vomiting in

Historical Highlights

The origin of the word nostril. This term is related to the common word "thrill." The Middle English *thrillen* originally meant to pierce. Nostril used to be spelled "nosethrill," a hole pierced in the nose.

We have been snorting things up our "nosethrills" for thousands of years. One of the first cultures to use the nose as an orifice for inserting medication was the Chinese. Chinese physicians in the eleventh century scraped the scabs off smallpox victims and crushed them into a powder. The physicians would then prescribe the powder to be snorted through a straw in order to protect their patients from developing smallpox.

Moving into the nineteenth century, the journal, *The Casket,* reported that snorting powdered moss scraped from decaying skulls would dispel headaches.

cases of poisoning and it has also been used to treat the dopamine deficiency associated with Parkinson's disease.

Men with Parkinson's disease also suffer from erectile dysfunction. In fact, the loss of erectile function occurs very early in the course of Parkinson's disease (PD), even before they present with the classic findings of this degenerative neurologic disease— tremor, slowness of movement (bradykinesia) and rigidity.

As soon as L-dopa (the precursor to dopamine) was discovered as a treatment for Parkinson's disease in 1967, physicians, nurses and family members couldn't help but notice that quite a few patients who used it had erections as a side effect. At the time this side effect was mentioned with a nudge and a wink, while the possibility of using L-dopa as a treatment for the embarrassing malady known as impotence wasn't even entertained by self-respecting researchers or clinical physicians.

The drug seligiline, also known as Eldepryl, was introduced in 1990. Its mechanism of action prolonged the effect of dopamine in the brain and gave patients with Parkinson's disease a needed boost—especially in the movement department, but also in the erection department. Once again, researchers overlooked its potential as a treatment for the male with your basic, everyday, run-of-the-mill impotence problem. And, once again, the nudge and a wink, elbow in the ribs, knee slap, and jokes about erections occurring as a side effect of the drug were made with great abandon.

There was even a commercial pornographic movie named "El Dopa." In fact, when the sales force for seligiline met to learn more about the drug to promote it to physicians and health care organizations, actors played the roles of Senor El Dopa and the lovely Senorita Eldepryl. They bantered on about the amusing side effect of Eldepryl with the closing remarks as follows:

A forlorn El Dopa: "I must leave you, I am starting to fade."

Senorita Eldepryl looked up and replied: "You don't have to leave. I can enhance your potency."

(The audience roars…the lights fade… the curtains close.)

Back to the second drug approved for erectile dysfunction—Uprima. When the first 50 volunteers with erectile dysfunction tested the drug, it worked and of course, that was the *good* news. Uprima boosted dopamine in the area of the brain controlling erections. The *bad* news: It also boosted dopamine in the vomiting center of the brainstem. The combination of erections with vomiting doesn't conjure up a warm, fuzzy, cuddly, sexy feeling in any of the parties involved.

Back to the drawing board…. After the first trials, Uprima was sent back to the research lab and was re-formulated to solve the vomiting problem. The results are as follows: Approximately 50 percent of the men who take it have erections firm enough for intercourse, and approximately 5 percent of the men taking the drug experience nausea, vomiting, dizziness, or sleepiness. Needless to say, this isn't the most popular treatment for erectile dysfunction.

Stay tuned for the next generation of drugs used for erectile dysfunction.

Take a snort to give "it" a boost. The FDA is currently evaluating a new nasal spray containing apomorphine that will promote an erection in less than 15 minutes, half the time it takes Viagra to do the same thing. Look for it in early 2004. The FDA has also approved a second-generation nitric oxide releasing drug—the son of Viagra, so to speak.

Panda perks from the Pfizer riser. Chinese zookeepers have contacted Pfizer Pharmaceuticals for doses of sildenafil (Viagra) for their male pandas held in captivity. It seems as if male pandas do not hold the world's record for sustaining an erection. In fact, 30 seconds is about average for the average male panda. Hardly long enough to maintain a robust panda population. So, the zookeepers have urgently requested Pfizer to help improve their chances of reproducing and increasing the population of this endangered species. It could work. Viagra is expected to improve their sexual endurance (wouldn't anything be better than 30 seconds?), and in turn, increase the chances of impregnating their partners. Stay tuned….

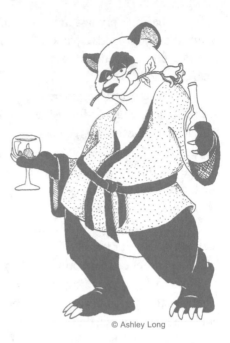

© Ashley Long

Viagra and saving the animals. The use of Viagra around the world has also reduced the poaching and slaughter of certain species for their body parts to be used as aphrodisiacs. Reindeer antlers and seal penises have been used in traditional impotence remedies; however, Viagra is cheaper than the killing of these animals for their parts and for what it's worth, Viagra is also more *effective* than a seal's penis or a reindeer's antler. A couple of researchers from the University of South Wales analyzed data on legally traded animals used in the traditional potions and lotions recommended for treating impotence. They found that in one year, antler sales fell from $700,000 to $200,000, and the number of seal penises sold dropped a whopping 50 percent—from 40,000 to 20,000.

A warning about recommending the herbal Viagra known as yohimbine. Yohimbine, from the bark of a West African tree, has long been described as a "male potency enhancer." The distributors of yohimbine have also described it as an herbal Viagra, however, buyer beware. It has not been effective as a sexual enhancer in men with normal sexual function, but it may have some effect in men with psychological erectile dysfunction. Studies in rats were quite promising—and in this case it's quite fortunate that human results don't mimic the results of rat studies. Male rats fed yohimbine were able to copulate 45 times in 15 minutes. The female rats in the study were not amused.

Unfortunately yohimbine has a few side effects that can send you straight to the emergency room, bypassing the bedroom. These include increased blood pressure, and numerous drug and food interactions (antidepressants known as the MAO inhibitors as well as chocolate, aged cheeses, beer, wine, nuts, and aged red meats). Patients also experience nervousness, anxiety, tachycardia, hypertensive crisis, and hallucinations.

Mesmer, Franz (1734-1815), was a Viennese physician who promoted a form of hypnotism in the eighteenth century commonly referred to as "mesmerism." During the early part of the eighteenth century the newly discovered properties of magnetism had become popular. Mesmer evolved a theory that a similar force could exercise a profound effect on the human body. This supposed force, known as "animal magnetism," purportedly could be transferred from one person to another. The practice of summoning and exerting this force, widely promoted by Dr. Mesmer, was a form of hypnotism, and thus, "to mesmerize" became a part of the language. Both Mesmer and mesmerism fell into disrepute when French authorities, commissioned to investigate Dr. Mesmer and his method, issued an unfavorable report.

The placebo effect. *Placebo* is the Latin word for "I shall please." Historically the term entered the world of medical terminology in the late eighteenth century and was used to *please* the patient, rather than *benefit* the patient. However, contrary to the initial use solely to assuage the patient's desire for a medication, numerous studies have shown that placebo actually confers significant benefit to many patients. Most health practitioners believe that the placebo effect has proven medical benefits and if properly utilized it can be an important component of a comprehensive and holistic treatment approach used by health practitioners.

Many conditions have been treated with what is now referred to as the placebo effect—mild to moderate pain, hypertension, depression, panic disorder, angina, degenerative joint disease and even warts. Up to 70 percent of depressed patients taking a placebo report an improvement in symptoms. When placebo was added to a heart failure regimen consisting of digitalis and a diuretic, patients improved considerably, compared to patients solely taking the digitalis and the diuretic alone.

Even telling a patient that they will get better has a significant impact on healing. A British study compared two groups of patients who had physical ailments but no specific diagnosis. Those in the first group were told their symptoms were not serious and they would improve in a short period of time. Patients in the second group were only told that the cause of their ailment was unclear. Two weeks later, 64 percent of the first group had improved compared to only 39 percent of the second group.

The power of positive thinking is at work here. When patients expect to improve, they have a better chance of recovering. When patients are told that a medication is going to help them they typically have a better response. People who are given an adult beverage that contains nary a drop of alcohol can feel and act intoxicated if they are told that the beverage contains booze.

Conditioned responses are also part of the placebo response. Remember our friends, Dr. Pavlov and his dogs? Pavlov sprinkled a powdered food substance on the tongues of dogs and rang a bell at the same time. The dog salivated. Powdered tongue, bell, salivation. Repeat. After a few applications, Pavlov would just ring the bell and the dog would salivate. Hence, the conditioned response. Patients with asthma have been shown to improve their symptoms by using an empty inhaler or even from hearing the sound of someone else using an inhaler. Patients on chemotherapy have been known to vomit as soon as they see their chemotherapy nurse.

Placebo therapy is most effective with diseases that have an emotional, stressful component, such as depression, pain, asthma, and hypertension. Taking the placebo can minimize the accompanying stress of the disease—blood pressure falls, cortisol levels decline, immunity improves, and pain is reduced.

The physician as placebo. Never underestimate the power of the "white lab coat." "He cures most successfully in whom the people have the most confidence." —Galen, second century B.C.

In other words, a confidence in the physician or other health care provider wearing tennis shoes and rag-tag hole-in-the-knees blue jeans just doesn't cut the mustard when it comes to instilling confidence. Stethoscopes, white coats, and prescriptions bolster confidence in the physician. One study showed that patients who were given a written prescription for exercise increased their physical activity to a greater extent than those given the same advice verbally.

Throughout the ages, warts have been especially susceptible to

Historical Highlights

In the mid-nineteenth century advocates of physical causes for mental illness recommended bloodletting, purging, cold-water immersion, and various tonics and medications (primarily opium and opium derivatives) as treatments. Others believed emotional disorders were caused by such problems as inappropriate mothering; it was thought impossible for patients to recover while remaining at home. Part of the treatment was to place the mentally ill patients in a mental asylum. To simplify management, many of these patients were restrained in straitjackets or manacles and chains.

the placebo effect. In fact, a German physician, Dr. Bruno Block, was a world famous wart-killing specialist in the 1920s. He had a wart-whacking machine complete with flashing lights and booming noises that beamed lethal "antiwart" rays in all directions. People flocked to his practice from all over Europe. He claimed to have "cured" hundreds of patients covered with thousands of warts. Heck, if it's the flashing lights and loud noises that zap warts, Las Vegas would be the wart-curing capital of the Western world.

Dr. Block's cure was quite sophisticated compared to that of Tom Sawyer and Huck Finn. According to Tom and Huck, all you had to do was:

"Go to the middle of the woods where there's a spunkwater stump and jest as it turns midnight you back up against the stump and jam your hands in it and say:

'Barleycorn Barleycorn, Injun meal shorts
Spunkwater, spunkwater SWALLER these warts.'"

Opium. Opium poppy seedpods found in Swiss lake dwellings may have been used for dulling the senses as far back as 4000 B.C. In 1020 B.C. Avicenna of Persia stated that opium is "the most powerful of all stupefacients."

Premarin vaginal cream and feminizing your husband. Premarin (estrogen) vaginal cream is inserted into the vagina in postmenopausal women as a treatment for vaginal dryness and other genitourinary conditions associated with menopause. The cream takes a few weeks to start to work. The cream has to kick start the glands that provide lubrication for the vagina and this might take three to five

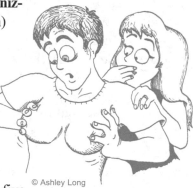
© Ashley Long

weeks. In the meantime, practitioners in the medical field advise their patients to use other forms of lubricants during this three to five week period. And, practitioners in the medical field stress to their patients that the Premarin vaginal cream should not be used as *the* lubricant. In other words, don't insert the cream, and immediately have sex with your husband. The vaginal cream can cross through the male urethra and the husband will receive a dose of estrogen. If this continues over a period of time your husband may be wearing a bigger bra that you do. This continued source of estrogen might enlarge his breasts, shrink his penis and testicles, and cause his voice to become a bit more high-pitched. *Yoo HOO, dahling!* He may also be fighting with you for the negligee on Friday night.

Rectal suppositories. Which end is up? Well, which end should be inserted first? The head of the suppository (the thick bulbous end) or the base (the skinny end)? Traditional insertion recommends that the apex has the privilege of entering the rectum first. However, a study with 100 subjects (60 adults and 40 children) compared apical vs. base insertion and found that 59 adults and 39 children preferred the base to be inserted first. Besides patient preference, two other advantages were found. One, there was no need to insert the finger into the rectal canal when the base was inserted first. Two, the incidence of expulsion (having it come right back at ya'), occurred only with apical insertion. The authors of the study (*Lancet,* Vol. 338, 1991) theorized that the arrangement of the muscles around the anal canal and rectum facilitate the insertion of the torpedo-shaped suppository with the base first. So, it's bottom's up instead of heads first.

> *Life—a sexually transmitted disease and the mortality rate is a hundred percent.*
> —R. D. Laing

Serotonin, also known as 5-hydroxytryptophan, was *initially* discovered in the gut in 1933 and it was referred to as enteramine. It was isolated in blood in 1948 and named as the serum factor. "Sero" meant that it was from serum. When serum factor was tested on blood vessels it caused them to have tonic constrictive activities, thus "tonin" was added to the "sero" and hence, the name Serotonin. Serotonin was found in the brain in 1953 and its location and general distribution in the brain were mapped by the mid 1960s. Serotonin in the brain alone has over 500,000 synapses. Serotonin has 16 different receptors at last count and has just as many functions. Serotonin makes you happy, gives you a sense of self-esteem, controls impulsive behaviors, makes you sleepy, makes you nauseated, makes you vomit, gives you diarrhea, and causes pain. She's just an all around kind of a gal with her positive and negative attributes.

Steroids and topical application. Here is a word of caution concerning the application of topical corticosteroids (hydrocortisone, for example). The absorption varies with body part application. If topical steroids are applied to the face and scalp there is a 5 to 10 times greater systemic delivery than if applied to the forearm. The genital skin, especially the scrotum, has up to 50 times more absorption that the forearm. The palms and the soles of the feet have one-fifth the absorption of the forearm. Steroid penetration is enhanced 5-to 100-fold if the skin is hydrated, so patients should be instructed to apply steroid cream after bathing when skin surfaces are still moist. Steroid penetration is also increased through inflamed skin. The third factor related to steroid absorption is the vehicle through which the steroid molecule is delivered. Ointments achieve better effects than creams or lotions of the same steroids.

> *Five minutes with Venus means a lifetime with Mercury.*
> —Anonymous

Syphilis and mercury. This quote describes the pleasures of sex (Venus, the goddess of love) combined with the misery of mercury for the treatment for syphilis in the sixteenth century. Mercury was the treatment of choice and was applied via a salve or in a fumigating chamber or both. Every practitioner of medicine (be it a surgeon, barber, quack, or midwife) had his or her own "special formula" containing mercury along with everything but the kitchen sink. Some mixed the mercury with pork fat, fresh butter, a touch of vinegar, a dash of myrrh, a milliliter of turpentine and sulfur, while others added live frogs, chicken's blood, snake venom, and a dash of human flesh to the blend.

Syphilitic patients would be slathered with this ointment, wrapped in hot towels and heavy blankets, and tossed in a hot tub, bath, or oven to bake. The theory behind the mercury mix combined with the heat application was that endless sweating and salivating would rid the body of the evil pox, (if it didn't kill you first). The mercury caused copious amounts of drooling. In fact, the treatment wasn't considered too successful if you didn't drool at least four pints on the first day. The usual length of treatment was 28 days. The biggest obstacle to treatment success was premature death. Most patients couldn't tolerate this torture and they died from heart failure, dehydration (not a surprise here), suffocation, and mercury poisoning. It wasn't a pretty sight.

Survivors of the mercury treatments didn't fare much better. They were deathly pale from bone marrow failure and anemia, they were toothless, hairless, and drooled uncontrollably. Needless to say they weren't hard to pick out of a crowd. So, you either died from syphilis or you died trying to cure it. The choice was all yours.

For those who refused the mercury "cure," other options included downing a bowl of ant's nest chowder, sticking earthworm plasters on their festering "poxes," or, my favorite, strapping a dead chicken to the penis. The infinite number of crude comments that can be made at this juncture is endless, so I will just zip it with a "no comment" through a clenched jaw.

Testosterone in clinical medicine. The clinical use of male secretions and sexual organs has its known origins in ancient Egyptian and Roman history. The Egyptians described the medicinal powers of the testicles and the Romans discussed the use of the donkey-penis and the honey-covered hyena penis as sexual fetishes. The ingestion of testis tissue was recommended for impotence as early as 1000 B.C. Testicular extracts were described as aphrodisiacs in A.D. 777-857.

In the late 1890s, Dr. Charles Edouard Brown-Sequard, a prominent French physiologist, extracted fluid from the testicles of dogs and guinea pigs and injected himself with the extract. He claimed that the injections not only improved his physical strength and mental prowess, but also relieved his constipation and most important of all, "lengthened the arc of his urine." Within a year of Brown-Sequard's claim of increased energy and virility, physicians from Bangkok to Bangor were giving testicular extract for just about everything from cancer to cholera, dementia to dysentery, seizures to sexual dysfunction.

Another well-known French physiologist of that same era, Dr. Claude Bernard, also proposed the use of "internal secretions" to enhance or restore the function of various glandular structures. Brown-Sequard's use of "internal secretions" initiated the era of hormone replacement therapy. These "internal secretions" were given a name in 1905—hormones.

Most of the "internal secretion" replacement therapy involved the extraction of fluids from the appropriate animal tissues for clinical use. In the late 1800s, two Austrian researchers, a physiologist and a physician, investigated whether testicular extracts could increase muscle strength and possibly improved performance. They injected themselves with a liquid extract from a bull's testicles and then measured the strength in their middle fingers. (Did they measure the strength of their middle fingers as a gesture to someone who annoyed them? Or were they lifting weights with the middle fingers? This was not mentioned in the text of the research abstract.) They published a paper in 1896 and concluded that the "orchitic"(orchi = testes) extract had improved both muscle strength and muscle conditioning. They recommended that the "training of athletes offers an opportunity for further research in this area and for a practical assessment of our experimental results."

At the same time (1890s), Russian chemists were studying a semen extract and its effects on the oxygen-carrying capacity of red blood cells. They observed that this extract caused the pH of blood to become more alkaline and this in turn increased the oxygen-carrying capacity of the red blood cells.

In 1931 it took 15,000 liters of policemens urine to synthesize 15 mg of testosterone. A major breakthrough was reported in 1935. Dr. Adolf Butenandt, a German biologist, successfully synthesized The Big T in the laboratory. This was hailed as "medical dynamite," "sexual TNT." Testosterone was officially recognized as the primary hormone produced by the testicles thanks to Dr. B. It only took four years for Adolf to walk up to the podium in Stockholm to receive his Nobel Prize for his discovery.

Since 1935 testosterone and its primary derivatives, the anabolic-androgenic steroids, have been the source of continued controversy. By 1937 human clinical trials were underway. By 1940, athletes and body-builders began self-administering testosterone propionate via injection and taking oral doses of methyl testosterone to increase muscle mass and intensify training programs. This "illegitimate" use of testosterone was recognized as the norm for many years and physicians routinely prescribed it to athletes for its "anabolic" (to build up) properties.

"Legitimate" uses of testosterone have also been recognized for over 50 years. Hormonal replacement therapy for primary testicular failure (medical or surgical) is a routine practice as is testosterone replacement in various congenital syndromes involving testosterone deficiency, such as Klinefelter's syndrome.

Testicular transplants of human and animal tissue began in 1912 in Philadelphia. Two physicians successfully transplanted a human testicle into a patient suffering from "dysfunctional sex glands." They reported a "technical" success but no mention was made of a "functional success." One year later a Chicago physician published a report detailing the transplantation of one testicle from a healthy donor into a patient that had lost both testicles. No mention was made as to how that patient lost both testicles, only that he received a donor testicle. Four days later the patient reported a "strong erection accompanied by marked sexual desire." In fact, he insisted on leaving the hospital, against medical advice, to satisfy his desire. No mention was made as to how far he had to travel to complete his mission. The patient did report back two years later that his sexual prowess was still intact.

Perhaps the most infamous testicular transplant surgeon was Dr. Leo L. Stanley, resident physician of San Quentin Federal Prison. In 1918 he began transplanting testicles from fresh donors. Hmmm. You might wonder who would qualify as a "fresh donor" in this instance. It just so happened that the fresh donors were recently executed prisoners. Dr. Stanley had a never-ending supply of prison inmate recipients of various ages and stages of sexual dysfunction. He reported marked improvement of sexual function in all recipients. When Dr. Stanley ran out of fresh donors he substituted ram, goat, deer, and boar testicles, which he claimed worked just as well as the human testicles. He became famous for treating just about any and every ailment with testicular replacement. Patients received testicles for senility, asthma, epilepsy, diabetes, tuberculosis, paranoia, gangrene, and even impotence.

Clinical uses of testosterone. Clinical uses of testosterone today are not quite as broad as they were in the early twentieth century. Nor do we get our supply of testicles from "fresh donors" from the penitentiary. The past and present uses of testosterone products (a.k.a. anabolic steroids) include replacement therapy for low or absent testosterone production, the treatment of wasting syndromes including HIV and AIDS, increasing libido in postmenopausal females, boosting appetites and a sense of well-being in AIDS and cancer patients, suppressing the symptoms of endometriosis, treating osteoporosis in older men, treating cognitive dysfunction, and interestingly enough using the hormone as a male contraceptive.

The most frequent and accepted therapy is the use of testosterone replacement for men with primary and secondary testicular failure. It may also be used to treat impotence in patients with low testosterone levels.

The use of testosterone to treat wasting syndromes associated with chronic debilitating illnesses began after World War II. Androgen supplements were used to treat the emaciated survivors of the Nazi concentration camps as well as soldiers suffering from burns, extensive surgery and battle injuries. Most recently, anabolic steroids have been effectively used to treat the weakness and muscle wasting that accompanies HIV, AIDS, and terminal cancer. This group of patients experience an improvement in appetite, sense of well-being, and an improvement in strength and an increase in muscle mass.

Prior to bone marrow transplants and the discovery and synthesis of synthetic erythropoietin, anabolic steroids were used to increase the production of red blood cells in patients with severe anemias.

In the past, women with conditions resulting from estrogen excess were treated with testosterone derivatives. Changing the hormonal environment in the woman with metastatic breast cancer resulted in tumor regression in some patients. The same rationale was applied to the treatment of endometriosis, a condition exacerbated by excess estrogen. The masculinizing side effects were a major drawback. These include a husky voice, facial hair, receding hairline, chest and back hair, and an enlarged clitoris. Pretty. Testosterone therapy is rarely used today for these conditions because of newer and more effective therapies.

A current use of testosterone in women combines a small amount of testosterone with estrogen in postmenopausal females with a loss of libido. This combination, known as Estratest, combines a dose of testosterone known as methyltestosterone, with estrogen. It provides a significant boost in libido as well as a boost in energy and a sense of well-being. Once it kicks in *look out!* She'll go from a lackluster libido to a wanton woman with no smooth transition in between. So when she makes the call, even if you're in a high-powered business meeting, you might want to excuse yourself and scurry on home.

The use of testosterone as a male contraceptive has interesting implications. High doses of exogenous (from the outside of the body, or synthetic) testosterone send an inhibitory message to the hypothalamic-pituitary axis. This message tells the hypothalamus and the pituitary gland that the body has adequate testosterone levels and that there is no need to release hormones to stimulate the production of testosterone. The hypothalamus responds by reducing the output of gonadotropin-releasing hormone and the pituitary responds by reducing the output of luteinizing hormone. Low levels of both centrally produced hormones decrease the production of testosterone by the testicle with the subsequent reduction of sperm production. The question is? Does it reduce the sperm production to *zero?* A zero number would be the only acceptable birth control method. You realize that even if *one* sperm is produced it will swim across the Pacific Ocean to fertilize an egg.

As a brief digression, the above scenario is also responsible for the side effects produced by anabolic steroids taken by athletes to boost their performance. When the athlete takes these drugs for strength and muscle building the feedback to the hypothalamus and pituitary turn off his own testosterone production and levels plummet. This explains the reproductive side effects of anabolic steroid use by athletes. They have decreased libido, decreased sperm counts, and a decrease in the size of the penis and testicles.

The studies using testosterone in the older male population are currently ongoing. Male testosterone levels rarely fall as dramatically as female estrogen levels with ovarian failure at menopause. Male testosterone levels at age 65 are approximately 50 percent lower than the levels of a 25-year-old male; however, the clinical effects appear to be negligible as compared to the lack of estrogen in the postmenopausal female. Nonetheless, the reduction of testosterone may contribute to a slower sexual response and a decreased libido, a reduction in orgasmic potential, reduced lean muscle mass, and a possible reduction in cognitive function concerning spatial orientation and word memory. Testosterone replacement may have beneficial effects on all of the above parameters.

Tobacco hasn't always been given such a bad rap as a cause of multi-system disease. In fact, in the early 1800s it was used therapeutically as a muscle relaxant. A strong cigar was introduced into the patient's rectum in order to relax the muscles prior to surgery. Some physicians dispensed with the formality of placing the cigar in the rectum and would either blow smoke directly into the rectum or inject tobacco distillates into the blood. And you wondered where the origin of the term "Smokin'" came from.

Vaccines—a bit of history. In the eleventh century Chinese doctors were intentionally infecting their patients with a mild form of smallpox, in hopes that it would confer immunity. It was called "sowing" or "buying" the pox. The Chinese physicians "sowed the pox" by making a powder from the dried scabs of victims and then having their healthy patients inhale the powder through straws. In other societies physicians made small incisions into the skin and rubbed the powder directly into the wound. This method of inoculation was called "ingrafting" and was popular in the seventeenth and eighteenth centuries in Europe and Great Britain. The smartest woman of all was Catherine the Great of Russia. She imported a British physician to vaccinate her entire court and she paid him an outrageous fee to do so.

Quarantine as a treatment for infectious disease. Quarantine as a treatment and prevention for infectious disease dates back to 1423 when Venice began confining sailors aboard ships at anchor for 40 days to protect the city from plaque. Quarantine is derived from the Latin word *quaresma,* meaning "forty."

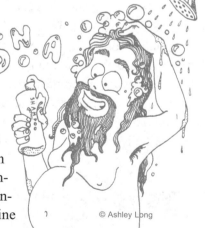

Vaccines via shampoos. DNA vaccines are becoming the "in" things these days in the field of immunology. Researchers at Stanford University have discovered that a simple solution of hepatitis B DNA and water applied to the skin of a mouse can induce a better immune response than the traditional intramuscular injection of the vaccine

© Ashley Long

Live a Little, Laugh a Lot

series. The gene from the DNA vaccine is transferred to the DNA of the hair follicle. The hair follicle subsequently produces the protein coded for by the gene. Tissue macrophages recognize the foreign protein, engulf the protein, and present it to the specific cells of the immune system. The subsequent immune response produces antibodies to that foreign protein.

DNA vaccines have been called the "third revolution" in vaccine science. The first vaccines, more than 100 years ago, were based on injections of dead or weakened pathogens. In the "second revolution," during the past 20 years, scientists have immunized the masses with a single protein from the pathogen. The third revolution DNA vaccines extend the techniques of the second revolution. Instead of a single protein being used, scientists inject the gene that makes the immune-stimulating protein. This "gene" vaccine appears to stimulate the immune response more vigorously than injecting just the protein. If you are scratching your hairy head and wondering why this DNA vaccine produces an even greater immune response than injecting the immune-stimulating protein directly, you are not alone. Researchers are scratching their baldheads and wondering the same thing.

In fact, this entire scenario was stumbled upon accidentally. It had been the assumption for years by the scientific community that in order for a vaccine to work it had to be injected into the muscle, or directly into the blood. Researchers at Stanford University were attempting to demonstrate this long-held

A survey of 2,212 members of the International Conference of Symphony and Opera Musicians indicated that propranolol (Inderal) is to contemporary classical music as liquor was to bebop, LSD was to late-1960s rock, or marijuana is to reggae.
(Fishwein, M, Middlestadt, SE. *Medical problems among ICSOM musicians: Overview of a national survey.* Med Prob Perform Artists 1988; 3:1-8.)

assumption by injecting the traditional vaccine and comparing it to dripping the DNA vaccine onto the skin of a mouse. They were mystified when the dripped vaccine demonstrated a stronger response than the injected vaccine.

Subsequent experiments explained the new findings. The cells within the hair follicles take up and make the protein from the DNA-vaccine gene. This triggers the vigorous immune response mentioned previously. The reason is obvious now—the skin faces a constant barrage from infectious microbes; therefore it has evolved a means to efficiently generate an immune response. This explains why the DNA vaccine doesn't work on hairless mice—you need hair follicles to transfer the gene.

Researchers are also experimenting with a number of needle-free ways of administering these vaccines including nasal sprays, dermal patches, and edible vaccines to present the genetic material to the immune system.

Rethinking needle size for adult vaccines. Another consequence of our "growing" society just happens to affect the size of needles used for vaccination purposes. Vaccines are being given into *fat* tissue instead of muscle tissue. Since our society continues to gain weight, many of the standard immunization needles won't penetrate deep enough to hit a muscle. Subcutaneous fat tissue is less vascular than muscle tissue; hence the immune system doesn't stand much of a chance in recognizing the foreign substance and therefore is unable to mount an appropriate immune response to it. The standard 5/8-inch needle isn't long enough for about 17 percent of men and nearly 50 percent of women. How embarrassing is *that*? Ladies, we need to join Weight-Lifting 101 classes to build up our deltoids. For IM injections, use a 1-inch needle for average size adults, and a 1.5-inch needle for women over 200 pounds and men over 260 pounds. (*British Medical Journal* 2000; 321: 1237)

A remedy for the pain of childbirth. "For Sharpe & Dificult Travel in Women with child Take a Lock of Vergins haire on any Part of ye head, of half the Age of ye Woman in travill. Cut it very smale to fine Powder the take 12 Ant Eggs dried in an oven after ye bread is drawne or other wise make them dry & make them to powder with the haire, give this with a quarter of a pint of Red Cows milk or for want of it give it in strong ale wort." —Dr. Zeobabel Endecott of Salem, Massachusetts (1659)

P.S. Most women took this potion in the strong ale wort. Milk was scarce in those days, but there was plenty of alcohol to consume. Thank goodness. I doubt it was the hair of the virgin or the ant eggs that eased the pain of childbirth. Most likely it was the stiff shot of the strong ale.

Is it pathology or is it due to the aging process? As practitioners we want to avoid dismissing treatable pathology as simply a process of aging and we also want to avoid treating natural aging processes as though they are diseases. The latter scenario is particularly dangerous because the elderly are so vulnerable to side effects and iatrogenic (physician or treatment-induced) effects. A frequently quoted story captures the dilemma: A 102-year-old man complained to his physician about pain in his right knee. The physician dismissed it. "What can you expect at 102?" But the patient retorted, "My left knee is 102 years old too, and it doesn't hurt."

I was going to buy a copy of The Power of Positive Thinking, and then I thought, What the hell good would that do?
—Ronnie Shakes

*You don't stop laughing because you grow old,
you grow old because you stop laughing.*

Index

Live a Little, Laugh a Lot

Blood thinner
Dwight David Eisenhower 302
Blood transfusion
Safety 166
Blood vessels 40
Calcium channel blockers 292
Flu shots 178
Herpes 184
Hormonal fluctuations 38
Mosquito bits 197
Nitroglycerin 307
Platelets 39
Serotonin 317
Viagra 308
Bloodhound
Olfactory bulbs 47
Bobbitt zone 53
Body piercing 218
Boiled egg breath 38
Bone marrow
Blood cells 39
Bones
Carpal 252
Chest X-ray 270
Strength 43
Boredom 14
Borrelia burgdorferi 192
Botox 167
Botulinum 167, 168, 205
Botulism 167–168
Aluminum foil 168
E. Coli 0157:H7 205
Honey
Infants 168
Potatoes 168
Bovine breast 124
Brain 154
Alzheimer's 265
Cannabinoids 298
Cerebral cortex 45
Depression 73
Dreaming 44
Eldepryl 310
Elephant 46
Erectile dysfunction 309
Estrogen 72
Headache 267
Life after death 40

Mad cow disease 208
Metabolic activity 75
Neurons 39
Orbital frontal cortex 73
Roller coaster ride 54
Serotonin 317
Sexual identity 73–74
SOAP BRAIN MD 254
Tourette's syndrome 213
Whispering endearments 33
Brain attack
Viagra 308
Brain tumors
Librium 289
Brassieres 140
Breakbone fever 166
Breast
Breast-fed 22
Breast cancer 49, 71, 322
Alcohol 96
Antiperspirants 97
Dr. William Stewart Halsted 101
Historical perspective 97–98
Risk factors 100
Weight gain during pregnancy 120
Breast compression
Mammograms 100
Breast self exams 102
Breast size 100
Breast-feeding 103, 108
breast-feeding 212
Broccoli
Anti cancer agent 240
Chronic Sinusitis 27
Fiber 244
Bruno Block 315
Bubonic plague 169–171
Black Death 169
Dental pulp and DNA 170
Early plagues 171
Germ warfare 172
Recent cases 170
Bugs
Breakfast 172
Coffee mugs 162
Cuddly bears 176
Diarrhea 274
Good and bad 163

G

Gabriel Fallopius 175
Gallstones
  Long distance runners 17
Game Boys
  Oya yubi 30
Gardening 123
Gas 80, 198
  Basal flatal rate 42
  Belching 245
  Coccyx 32
  Distended abdomen 278
  Dr. Michael Levitt 33
  Gallbadder disease 279
  Healthy colon 244
  Hydrogen 27
  Sheep 47
  Ship High in Transport 12
Gastric by-pass 232
Gauze Pack
  Stuffy nose 26
Germs
  Coin laundry machines 178
Giardia 236, 237, 274
Giraffe 46
Global warming
  Health issues 195
  Infectious disease 194
Glove compartments 305
Glutathione Deficiency
  Chronic sinusitis 27
Gold dust 293
Golf 226
  Melanoma 261
Golf balls
  Pesticides 9
Golf courses 9
Great Plague 171
Group A Beta Hemolytic Strep 213
Group A beta hemolytic strep
  Children 262
Gum disease 110
Gut 9
Gyri 45

H

H. pylori 183, 240
Hair 40, 160, 322

Arsenic 18
Gallbladder disease 279
Hair color
  Employment opportunities 124
Hair follicle
  Vaccines in shampoo 325
Hair products 125
Hair spray
  Occupational hazard 17
Haircut 217
Hairdressers
  Birth defects 17
  MRSA 17
Haiti 216
Halcion 291
Hallmark greeting card
  Centenarians 36
Hamburgers 227, 237
  Spilled while driving 234
Hand washing
  Another reminder 179
  Artificial fingernails 180
  Physicians 182
  Restrooms 180
Hansen's disease 182
Hanson, G. Annauer. 182
Head butting
  HIV 182
Hearing Loss
  Airbags 37
  Decibels 37
Heart
  Aspirin 286
  C-reactive protein 49
  Chest X-ray 270
  Distended abdomen 278
  Elephant 46
  Elevated liver enzymes 275
  Extramarital affair 50
  Foxglove 304
  Laughter 28
  Leeches 300
  Mecury 318
  Nitroglycerin 307
  Placebo 314
  Rheumatic fever 255
  Saunas 18
  Smoking 56

Live a Little, Laugh a Lot

Monkey T (testosterone) 142
Monks
  Arthritis of the knees 14
Monthlies
  How many do we get 91
Morphine 262, 291
Morticians
  Tuberculosis 15
Mosquito
  Replication time 196
Mosquito bite 197, 201
Mosquitoes 196, 199
Motor vehicle accident 52
MRSA
  Hospital hairdresser 17
Mucus 44
Munchausen syndrome 205, 283
Murphy, Edward A.
  Murphy's Law 12
Muscle Strength
  Mental training 29
Muscle strength 264, 320
Museum of Menstruation 89
Myocardial infarction 49, 178, 269
  Deer hunters 18
  Dwight David Eisenhower 302
  Monday mornings 21
  New Year's Day 21
  Saunas 18
  Seasonal 21
  Shoveling snow 21
  Viagra 308
Myopia
  Refined starches 235

N

Nail biting 43
Nail trauma 43
Napoleon 18, 285
Natural feel condoms 175
Navel Piercing 190
Nazi 206, 249, 322
NEAT 229
Neck 54
  NFL football players 24
  Sleep apnea 24
Nephritis and septicemia 121
Nephrons 41

Nerves 197, 210, 280
  Cranial 253
  Impulses 39
  Optic 43
Neurons 39, 213
New Year's Day 53
  Myocardial infarction 21
Nidetch, Jean
  Weight Watchers 231
Night owl 46
Nitric oxide 308
  Erection 311
Nitroglycerin 306–307
  Glove compartment 305
Nitrous oxide
  Dental Workers 16
  Laughing gas 16
North Korea 214
Nose 177, 201, 218, 243, 310
  Bloodhound 47
  Chronic sinusitis 26
  Crying 69
  Estrogen 67
  Gauze packs 26
  Genitals 76
  Nosebleed 2
  Nosethrill 22
Nosebleed
  Menstruation 76
Nosethrills 310
Nostril 26, 310
NTG 306

O

Obese 229
Obesity 48
  Exercise 230
  Fast food in hospitals 245
  Reducing life span 230
  Surgery 232
  Virus 220
Occupational hazard
  Bronze Age metal workers 18
  Chimney sweep 15
  Church bell ringers 14
  Coroners 15
  Crematorium workers 15
  Dental Hygienists 16

APPENDIX
Answers to the "Quizzicles"

Huh? Quizzicles? A law professor was well known for his pop quizzes in his class on tax law. He told the students that they would have a series of these "easy" pop quizzes during the semester and one final test at the end. He would use a ridiculous "cutsie" name for the quizzes and call them "quizzicles." As he continued to give these over the course of a semester the students became increasingly agitated because the so-called "quizzicles" were annoying and also difficult. One woman finally raised her hand in frustration and screamed out: "If these pop 'quizzicles' are so damn easy, I can't wait to see your 'testicles!'" Anyway, here are the answers to your "quizzicles" from each chapter.

Chapter 4

This syndrome affects nearly 6 percent of all premenopausal women. It has numerous systemic manifestations including infertility, endometrial cancer, diabetes, and heart disease. In addition, women have male-pattern baldness and an overabundance of coarse, dark male-pattern hair distribution. Seventy-five years ago two French physicians described this condition as "the diabetes of bearded women." Name this syndrome.

Answer: Polycystic ovary syndrome or PCOS (prounounced 'pee-kos')

Chapter 6

This infectious disease is carried by a mosquito. One of the hallmarks of this disease is musculoskeletal pain so severe that it is sometimes referred to as "breakbone" fever. What is the name of this disease?

Answer: Dengue fever

Mycobacterium leprae, identified by the Norwegian bacteriologist G. Annauer Hansen, is an obligate intracellular parasite found exclusively in only two hosts. One of the hosts is the human and the second host is (you'll never guess it in 1 million years).
Answer: The armadillo.

Chapter 7

What animal is a natural host for *Giardia?* _____
Answer: The beaver.
Speaking of beavers, did you know that the beaver is a strict vegetarian and only eats the bark from hardwood trees, leaves, and plants?

Italy leads the world in the consumption of pasta with 61.7 pounds consumed per person per year. Guessing the number two country in the world consuming pounds of pasta might be a bit more difficult. Any guesses?
Answer: Venezuela with 27.9 pounds of pasta per person.

General Bibliography

Angiers, N. *Woman: An Intimate Geography.* (2000) Anchor Books, New York, NY.

Asimov, I. *Isaac Asimov's Book of Facts.* (1979) Wings Books, New York, NY.

Bancroft, B. *An Apple a Day: The ABCs of Diet and Disease.* (2001) WellWorth Publishing, Albuquerque NM.

Blum, D. *Sex on the Brain.* (1997) Penguin Group, New York, NY.

Biddle, W. *A Field Guide to Germs.* (1995) Anchor Books, New York, NY.

Bodmer, K, Fuchs, NK. *The Giant Book of Women's Health Secrets.* (1998) Soundview Publications, Atlanta GA.

Cartwright, FF. *Disease and History.* (1972) Dorset Press, New York, NY.

Douglas, PS. *Cardiovascular Health and Disease in Women.* (1993) WB Saunders, Philadelphia PA.

Elia, I. *The Female Animal.* Henry Holt and Company. (1988) New York, NY

Golub, S. *Periods: From Menarche to Menopause.* (1992) Sage Publications, Newbury Park, CA.

Greenfield, SA. *The Human Brain.* (1997) Perseus Books Group. New York, NY.

Haggard, HW. *Devils, Drugs and Doctors.* (1980) Charles Rivers Books, Boston, MA.

Haubrich, WS. *Medical Meanings: A Glossary of Word Origins.* (1984) Harcourt Brace Jovanovich, San Diego, CA.

Jones, KN. *Medical acronyms, eponyms, and mnemonics.* (1998) Wysteria, Long Island, NY.

Kiple, KF. *The Cambridge World History of Human Disease.* (1994) Cambridge University Press. Cambridge, UK.

Legato MJ. Gender-Specific Aspects of Human Biology for the Practicing Physician. (1997) Futura Publishing Company. Armonk, NY

Love, SM. *Dr. Susan Love's Hormone Book.* Random House, Inc. 1998. New York, NY.

Maines, RP. *The Technology of Orgasm.* (1999) The Johns Hopkins University Press. Baltimore, MD.

Moore, KL. *Before We Are Born.* (1989) W.B. Saunders, Philadelphia, PA.

Nathanielsz, P. *Life Before Birth.* (1992) W.H. Freeman and Company, New York, NY.

Nathanielsz, P. *The Prenatal Prescription.* (2001) Harper Collins Publishers, New York, NY.

Parsons, A. *Facts and Phalluses.* (1989) St. Martin's Press, NY.

Porter, R. *Madness: a brief history.* (2002) Oxford University Press, New York, NY.

Pool, R. *Eve's Rib.* (1994) Crown Publishers Inc. New York, NY

Sadler, TW. *Langman's Medical Embryology.* (2000) Lippincott, Williams & Wilkins. New York, NY.

Sloane, E. *The Biology of Women.* (1993) Delmar Publishers. Albany, NY

Sapolsky, RM. *The Trouble with Testosterone.* (1997) Scribner, New York, NY.

Tierno, PM. *The Secret Life of Germs.* (2001) New York, NY.

Walker, S. *A Dose of Sanity: Mind, Medicine, and Misdiagnosis.* (1996) John Wiley & Sons, New York, NY.

Warren, Carol A.B. *Midwives: Schizophrenic Women in the 1950s.* (1964) Rutgers University Press, New Brunswick.

Bibliography for Mnemonics for Mnemcompoops

CA—A Cancer Journal for Physicians, June 1997.

Gill, D, O'Brien, N. *Paediatric Clinical Examination.* 3rd edition. Churchhill Livingston 1998.

Jacob, GM, Palmer, RM. Tools for assessing the frail elderly. *Postgraduate Medicine* 1998; 104(1):135-53.

Ransom, J. The current management of acute pancreatitis. *Advances in Surgery* 1995; 28:93-112.

Johnston, DE. Special considerations in interpreting liver function tests. *American Family Physician* 1999; 59(8):2223-30.

Ashley Long

Ashley Long, whose cartoons appear in *Live a Little, Laugh a Lot*, as well as Barb's previous book, *An Apple a Day—The ABCs of Diet and Disease*, is a twenty-year-old artistliving in Rapids City, Illinois. She is attending the College for Creative Studies in Detroit, MI, where she is in her third year of studying traditional animation. Her animations have competed at the Kalamazoo Animation Festival International, and can also be seen in the short film *25 Ways to Die*. In the past , Ashley has been employed as an animator, illustrator, rubber stamp designer, intern, and teaching assitant 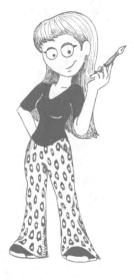 for an annual fine arts program. She is also serving as current president of the Secret Order of the Atomic Sea Monkeys animation club.

Contact Ashley at: *spatfat8@hotmail.com* or e-mail Wellworth Publishing.

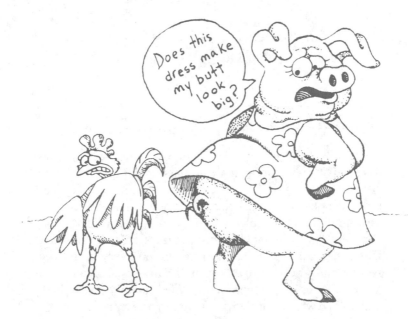

Don't Miss Barb's Book
An Apple a Day

An Apple a Day – the ABC's of Diet and Disease, written in Barb's usual witty style is sure to delight, amuse and educate. With quotes like the one above and chapters like **Chocolate, Chocolate and More Chocolate; Veggies, Vitamins and Viagra; Pizza Pasta and Prostate; Beans, Beans, the Musical Fruit** and 22 more, you are sure to find yourself chuckling, chortling and possibly guffawing at this priceless collection.

Only Irish coffee provides in a single glass all four essential food groups: alcohol, caffeine, sugar, and fat.

—Anonymous

An *Apple a Day* is receiving great reviews!

Written by Barb Bancroft, a health care professional who has been offering informative seminars since 1980, An Apple A Day: The ABC's Of Diet & Disease is a solid, understandable, easy-to-read reference written expressly to be understandable to non-professional general reader. Organized in encyclopedia-format A through Z, An Apple A Day offers solid, practical information on everything from Apples and Anorexia to the scam of Yam-based creams and a recipe for cold Zucchini Soup. Witty, heavily researched, and packed with so much information the reader is guaranteed to expand his or her knowledge on the good, the bad, and the ugly of foods and nutrition. Of special note are the entries dealing with food-borne illnesses. An Apple A Day is highly recommended for personal and community library health care reading lists and reference collections.

MidWest Book Review

$22 plus $4 shipping
Order form on last page